Davis's PA Exam Review
Focused Review for the PANCE and PANRE

Money-Back Guarantee

If you are a graduate of a Physician Assistant program accredited in the United States, take the PANCE and/or PANRE examination for the first time, and do not pass after using Davis's PA Exam Review: Comprehensive Guide to PANCE and PANRE Exams, return the book and accompanying CD to F.A. Davis Company, Customer Service, 404–420 North 2nd Street, Philadelphia, PA 19123. *Enclose your original receipt of purchase for the book and a copy of both your official test results notification and your certificate of graduation.* We will refund the price you paid for the book. If you have questions, please call 1-800-323-3555.

Davis's PA Exam Review
Focused Review for the PANCE and PANRE

Morton A. Diamond, MD, FACP, FACC, FAHA
Professor and Medical Director
Nova Southeastern University
Fort Lauderdale, Florida

F. A. Davis Company • Philadelphia

F. A. Davis Company
1915 Arch Street
Philadelphia, PA 19103
www.fadavis.com

Copyright © 2008 by F. A. Davis Company

Copyright by F. A. Davis Company. All rights reserved. This product is protected by copyright. No part of it may be reproduced, stored in a retrieval system, or transmitted in any form or by any means, electronic, mechanical, photocopying, recording, or otherwise, without written permission from the publisher.

Printed in the United States of America

Last digit indicates print number: 10 9 8 7 6 5 4 3 2 1

Publisher: Margaret Biblis
Acquisitions Editor: Andy McPhee
Sr. Developmental Editor: Jennifer A. Pine

As new scientific information becomes available through basic and clinical research, recommended treatments and drug therapies undergo changes. The author(s) and publisher have done everything possible to make this book accurate, up to date, and in accord with accepted standards at the time of publication. The author(s), editors, and publisher are not responsible for errors or omissions or for consequences from application of the book, and make no warranty, expressed or implied, in regard to the contents of the book. Any practice described in this book should be applied by the reader in accordance with professional standards of care used in regard to the unique circumstances that may apply in each situation. The reader is advised always to check product information (package inserts) for changes and new information regarding dose and contraindications before administering any drug. Caution is especially urged when using new or infrequently ordered drugs.

Library of Congress Cataloging-in-Publication Data

Diamond, Morton A.
 Davis's PA exam review : focused review for the PANCE and PANRE/Morton A. Diamond.
   p. ; cm.
 Includes index.
 ISBN-13: 978-0-8036-1873-2
 ISBN-10: 0-8036-1873-5
 1. Physicians' assistants—Examinations, questions, etc. 2. Physician Assistant National Certifying Exam—Study guides. I. Title. II. Tittle: PA exam review.
 [DNLM: 1. Physician Assistants—Examination Questions. 2. Certification—Examination Questions. W 18.2 D5377d 2008]
 R697. P45D53 2008
 610.73'72069076—dc22
                                                                                          2008009994

Authorization to photocopy items for internal or personal use, or the internal or personal use of specific clients, is granted by F. A. Davis Company for users registered with the Copyright Clearance Center (CCC) Transactional Reporting Service, provided that the fee of $.10 per copy is paid directly to CCC, 222 Rosewood Drive, Danvers, MA 01923. For those organizations that have been granted a photocopy license by CCC, a separate system of payment has been arranged. The fee code for users of the Transactional Reporting Service is: 8036–1873–5/08 + $.10.

In gratitude for their everlasting love

Louise
Regine, David, Michele, Laura,
Yael, Shira, Aviva

I thank Andy McPhee, Acquisitions Editor, and Jennifer Pine, Developmental Editor, at F.A. Davis Company for their support, guidance, and bonhomie.

Foreword

Recently a new physician assistant (PA) graduate of my program replied to a question about her preparation for the Physician Assistant National Certifying Examination (PANCE) by saying that she bought "every review text I could find." Not a surprising answer, given the importance of the examination to her career as a PA, and not surprising that she was able to find a number of review texts on the market. So what makes this text different?

Morton Diamond, a PA educator since 1994 and previously a practicing cardiologist, has constructed a unique and highly effective system that reviews medical concepts while at the same time teaches critical thinking. Rather than taking a body system approach he splits his book into two sections, the second building off the first.

In the first section, *Essentials,* he poses specific clinical scenarios and questions using a multiple-correct answer methodology. This approach allows for specific, detailed feedback on the range and depth of one's knowledge. The likelihood of answering the questions accurately just by guessing is significantly reduced using this method because the test-taker must select the correct *combination* of answers. Further, this method avoids the "one right answer," lower-order mentality so antithetical to the real world of medicine.

Answers in the text are provided alongside specific teaching points central to understanding the material. This approach ensures the integration of key concepts into the review of each subject. He also provides body system classification labels so that students can focus on the content they most need to review.

The second section, *Performance,* takes a more traditional approach to questions, with single correct answers for each, just as one would encounter on the PANCE and PANRE. However, even in this section, the correct answer is keyed back to its earlier discussion in *Essentials,* an approach that provides excellent testing as well as critical review.

Included with every book is a CD-ROM with even more questions, none of which are repeated in the book. The testing software on the CD-ROM allows users to take practice tests using a large pool of questions from a variety of topic areas or a smaller pool of questions from specific topic areas. Highly flexible and customizable, the testing software adds one more tool to the test-taker's arsenal of exam preparation weapons.

Dr. Diamond seems to understand exactly what a new graduate PA needs to know, as well as what practicing PAs need to know to recertify and remain in practice. New graduates and recertifying PAs will find this book-and-software package an invaluable tool in preparing for their next, critical examination.

DANA SAYRE-STANHOPE, EDD, PA-C
Associate Professor and Director
Physician Assistant Program Emory University School of Medicine
Atlanta, Georgia
Former Chair of the Accreditation Review Commission on Education
for the Physician Assistant

Reviewers

Anna M. Choo, MD, JD
Resident Physician
Department of Physical Medicine
  and Rehabilitation
Emory University Hospital
Atlanta, Georgia

Tom Colletti, MPAS, PA-C
Assistant Consulting Professor
Physician Assistant Program
Duke University School of Medicine
Durham, North Carolina

Katherine M. Erdman, MPAS, PA-C
Assistant Professor
Physician Assistant Program
Baylor College of Medicine
Houston, Texas

Richard Gicking, MD, FACP
Department of Medicine
Emanuel Hospital
Portland, Oregon

Diana Kharbat, DO
Resident Physician
Department of Physical Medicine
  and Rehabilitation
Emory University Hospital
Atlanta, Georgia

Naghmeh Khodai, MD
Resident Physician
Obstetrics/Gynecology
Rush University Medical Center
Chicago, Illinois

Adam J. Kinninger, DO
Intern
Osteopathic Medicine
St. Vincent Mercy Hospital
Toledo, Ohio

Clara LaBoy, PA-C, MS
Assistant Professor
Physician Assistant Program
Pacific University
Forest Grove, Oregon

Mary Ann Laxen, PA-C, MAB
Director
Physician Assistant Program
University of North Dakota
Grand Forks, North Dakota

Allison A Morgan, MPA, PA-C
Instructor
Department of Physician Assistant
Duquesne University
Pittsburgh, Pennsylvania

John Tobias Musser, MD
Resident Physician
Physical Medicine & Rehabilitation Residency
  Program
Department of Rehabilitation Medicine
Emory University School of Medicine
Atlanta, Georgia

Manali Indravadan Patel, MD, MPH
Resident Physician
Internal Medicine Residency Program
Stanford University School of Medicine
Stanford, California

Tammy Dowdell Ream, MPAS, PA-C
Coordinator of Clinical Education
Physician Assistant Program
Texas Tech University Health Sciences Center
Midland, Texas

John M. Schroeder, PA-C, JD
Associate Professor
Department of Physician Assistant Studies
Idaho State University
Pocatello, Idaho

Erica Young, PA-C
Physician Assistant
Correctional Managed Care
The University of Texas Medical Branch
Galveston, Texas

Kevan Zipin, MD
Resident
Emergency Medicine
Lincoln Medical and Mental Health Center
Bronx, New York

Student Reviewers

Abraham Balsamo
University of New Mexico
Albuquerque, New Mexico

Angelica Clark
Jefferson College of Health Sciences
Roanoke, Virginia

Jennifer Crook
University of Kentucky
Lexington, Kentucky

Tamar Dragon
Barry University
Miami Shores, Florida

Erin Duhaime
Stony Brook University
Stony Brook, New York

Kent Ellsworth
Idaho State University
Pocatello, Idaho

Lindsay Fisher
Marquette University
Milwaukee, Wisconsin

Kristen Frank
Drexel University
Philadelphia, Pennsylvania

Van Treia Gross
University of Maryland Eastern Shore
Princess Anne, Maryland

Ilyas Gutale
University of Maryland Eastern Shore
Princess Anne, Maryland

Kate Hartman
Idaho State University
Pocatello, Idaho

Sara Kennedy
Stony Brook University
Stony Brook, New York

Katie Machurik
University of Florida
Gainesville, FL

Stacy Montz
Loma Linda University
Loma Linda, California

Maryam Mottaghian
Stony Brook University
Stony Brook, New York

Richard Nellis
Des Moines University
Des Moines, Iowa

Kristi Posey
Baylor College of Medicine
Houston, Texas

Travis Randolph
University of Florida
Gainesville, Florida

Katey Reed
University of Florida
Gainesville, Florida

Courtney Simas
Kings College
Wilkes-Barre, Pennsylvania

Lee Ann Simmons
South College
Knoxville, Tennessee

Lauren von Almen
Drexel University
Philadelphia, Pennsylvania

The Author

Morton A. Diamond, MD, FACP, FACC, FAHA is a clinical cardiologist with nearly four decades' experience in the education of physician assistant students and medical students. Since 1994 he has been the full-time Medical Director of the Nova Southeastern University Physician Assistant Program in Ft. Lauderdale, Florida.

Dr. Diamond has extensive experience in medical test-writing and is considered to be a skilled and prolific writer of test questions. He has published many articles in peer-reviewed medical journals and has written chapters in medical textbooks. He is frequently invited to present lectures at state and national medical meetings.

Preface

This unique book promotes success on national Physician Assistant (PA) certifying examinations by employing a novel and highly efficient learning structure. The book is organized differently than any other PANCE/PANRE review book on the market, and it's organized that way to better help you pass those examinations. You'll find that the book is divided into two sections, Essentials and Performance.

Essentials is composed of didactic test items designed to enhance your knowledge. Items are constructed to enable the PA or PA student to compare and contrast medical data. Therefore, many test items in Essentials have *more than one* correct answer. Multiple correct answers force the test-taker to think more deeply. Each item in Essentials is followed by a succinct exposition called *You Should Know*. Each *You Should Know* provides key information critical to your understanding of the material.

You should consider Essentials as a bridge to Performance, the section of the book in which the medical knowledge base is tested through patient vignettes and accompanying test items. Performance is intended to give you a sense of the actual certifying examination. Each Performance item is linked (see **Performance Answer section**) to one or more specific test items in Essentials. Like the actual PANCE and PANRE, there is only *one best answer* to each test item in Performance.

No Logical Order

Davis's PA Exam Review is intentionally not structured in a logical order. Specifically, test items are not colligated by organ system, such as cardiovascular and endocrine, nor are they compiled by task, such as pathophysiology and clinical therapeutics. The chaotic order of test items in the book mimics the certifying examination and forces you to maintain an agile, fast-moving mind so you can move quickly and effectively from, say, a pediatric item to a preventive medicine item to a pharmacology item.

The book strives to present an equal distribution of items in the knowledge and skill areas being tested by the exams. These areas include history taking and physical examination, using laboratory and diagnostic studies, formulating most likely diagnoses, clinical interventions, clinical therapeutics, health maintenance, and applying scientific concepts.

Test Item Breakdown

Test items related to disorders by organ systems will be generally formulated as follows:

- 30% to 35% of the items relate to cardiovascular or pulmonary disorders
- 15% to 20% of the items relate to musculoskeletal or gastrointestinal disorders
- 20% to 25% of the items relate to EENT, reproductive, endocrine, or neurological disorders
- 20% to 25% of the items relate to psychiatric, genitourinary, dermatological, or hematological disorders, or infectious diseases

These percentage breakdowns roughly approximate the breakdown used for actual certifying examinations.

Advantages

If you've examined other PANCE/PANRE review books, you no doubt know that their test items offer only one correct answer. For instance, a review book might have a test item on atrial fibrillation in which diltiazem is the correct response. Yet in the patient with atrial fibrillation, slowing of the ventricular response is an essential element in treatment. Several medications may thus be used, including verapamil, diltiazem, propranolol, and digoxin. In no way does a test item requiring only one correct answer probe the test taker's ability to define the proper medication in a specific clinical setting, such as atrial fibrillation in a patient with heart failure.

This book, on the other hand, probes your knowledge in depth. It helps you to think critically and respond clinically, which the PANCE and PANRE both require.

You have undoubtedly found as well that other exam review books provide medical information *after* a test item has been answered. In contrast, this book enriches your information base in Essentials, well before you engage the test items in Performance. It is educationally more effective to inform first and, thereafter, to test, rather than to initially test and then, later, offer an explanation.

Last and most important, you will find that the test items here mirror exactly the format and structure of test items in actual certifying examinations. The author is a veteran item writer for PA certifying examinations and has taken great pains in crafting the test items in this book and CD-ROM to fit the items you will actually encounter on your examination.

About the CD-ROM

The CD-ROM that accompanies the book contains an electronic test bank in the popular and flexible test-generating software Wimba Tutor. With this self-paced testing and teaching software, you can choose from the available bank of test items by specifying areas to be tested. For instance, you can choose to be tested on just cardiovascular items, neurological and pulmonary items, or any combination of body system chapters.

The CD-ROM contains a test bank of more than 650 test items. After a test is graded, the score shows the test items broken down by chosen categories. That way you can identify weak areas and then focus on them in your studies.

Preparing for the Exam

If you are preparing for the Physician Assistant National Certifying Exam (PANCE), you already know that the test is a milestone in your Physician Assistant career. You have a sense of pride and accomplishment for having successfully completed rigorous academic training. PANCE is the final hurdle before you fulfill your bright promise of service, commitment, and caring.

If you are preparing for the Physician Assistant National Recertifying Exam (PANRE), you are seeking recertification that will demonstrate your having the requisite knowledge to meet the standard of your profession. Success in PANRE affords you the satisfaction of knowing you are a member of an elite medical profession that sets recertification standards.

Either way, you will want to read through this special section. It covers key test-taking tips for these examinations and also highlights exactly how test-item writers—the people who made the test you are about to take—craft questions, answers, and distractors. (See *What Experienced Test Writers Do*.) The more you know about how test items are built, the better prepared you will be to answer each item correctly.

Tips for Success

To pass either the PANCE or PANRE, you will need to prepare wisely, develop clear and efficient test-taking strategies, and know what to expect on test day.

Preparing Wisely

Before you do anything else, visit the National Commission on Certification of Physician Assistants (NCCPA) Web site at www.nccpa.net/. It offers information on test eligibility requirements, registration information, examination content blueprint, sample questions, and other important guidelines concerning the PANCE and PANRE. In addition, make sure to go through the demo (www.nccpa.net/EX_practiceexam.aspx). It explains much about the testing environment and test-taking software.

Read the NCCPA Content Blueprint, and learn as much as you can about the diseases and disorders listed. Use this book and accompanying CD-ROM for enriching your information base and practicing your test-taking skills.

For instance, you can practice your time-management skills by selecting a number of questions and then giving yourself an average of 1 minute per question to respond. By taking timed tests, you can become comfortable working under actual test-taking conditions.

Just Before Test Day

Make sure that you get to the test site on time. If you will be traveling to an unfamiliar location, obtain directions to the site. Then make a test drive before the day of the test. Remember to bring the directions with you on exam day.

If you live a considerable distance from the test site, arrive the day before the exam and stay overnight in the area. You will need a good night's rest to ensure your being as relaxed as possible.

Do not cram the night before taking the test. You need rest at this point, not more study. Bring a small snack with you for refreshment during break periods.

Test-taking Strategies

Here are a few strategies to employ when taking the test.

- Read each question carefully. Be aware of words and phrases such as *indicated, contraindicated, preferred initial* (therapy), and *except*. *Except* questions are generally rare, but be alert for their appearance nonetheless.
- Read all responses (*A* through *E*) before making your decision. Try to systematically exclude responses you know are incorrect.
- Do not spend an excessive amount of time on a single question. If you find that you have spent 2 minutes on a question, it is probably best to flag that question and return to it later, in the block-time period.

Exam Day

You should arrive at least 30 minutes before your test is scheduled to begin. If you arrive late, you may have to forfeit your breaks or pay a late fee to reschedule the examination.

Upon arrival at the test center you will present your scheduling permit. You must be prepared to show two forms of identification, including a driver's license or passport. Both must be original and valid (not expired). No one is permitted to take the examination without the permit and personal identification. Refer to NCCPA website for more details related to identification.

You are not allowed to bring personal belongings into the testing room. Examples of prohibited personal property include book bags, handbags, brimmed hats, books, notes, study materials, watches, electronic devices, and food or beverages. A locker will be assigned for storage of these items.

Staff members at the testing center will provide instructions to assist in use of the computer equipment. You will have the opportunity to complete a brief tutorial before starting the formal testing session. The examination will be observed by testing center staff members who will use audiovisual monitors and recording equipment.

Examination Structure

PANCE and PANRE examinations are administered in blocks. The PANCE consists of six blocks, each having 60 multiple-choice test items (see "Parts of a Test Item"), for a total of 360 test items. You will have 60 minutes to complete each block, a timeframe that represents an average of 1 minute per question.

PANRE consists of five blocks, each having 60 multiple-choice test items, for a total of 300 test items. You will have 60 minutes to complete each block, a time frame that represents an average of 1 minute per question.

In both PANCE and PANRE, test items may be answered in any order within a block. You may review questions, and answers may be changed within a block during the time allotted for that block. You will have a total of 45 minutes for breaks between blocks. You are solely responsible for managing your break time, so manage it well.

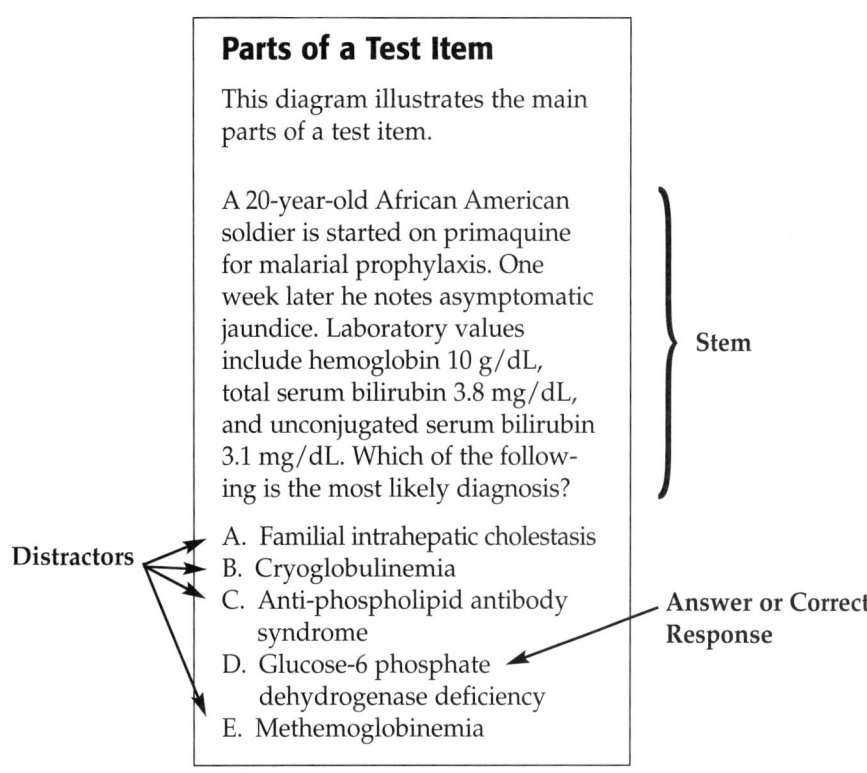

What Experienced Test Writers Do

Experienced test-writers commonly use certain terms or phrases for consistency and clarity in presentation. Your familiarity with those terms or phrases will make you more comfortable during the exam. Here are five key tips for understanding what experienced test writers do and what you can learn from it.

Tip #1: Worry Not About the Small Stuff

Item writers, when constructing a clinical vignette, typically write that the patient *has* a symptom rather than *complains of* a symptom. For example, an item stem might read, "A 52-year-old man has a 1-hour history of chest pressure," or "A 42-year-old woman has a 3-week history of nausea and weight loss." You should understand that *has* is essentially equivalent to *complains of*.

Here's another example. In clinical vignettes, item writers often use the phrase *Examination shows* when describing physical signs of a disease or disorder. For instance, you might see something like "Examination shows the apical impulse to be in the fifth intercostal space," or "Examination shows hyperpigmentation in the skin creases." Yes, there are other ways to say the same thing, but PANCE and PANRE item writers tend to use just this one.

Tip #2: Differentiation

Item writers generally construct items that force the test candidate to clinically distinguish between two diseases. They tend to use the phrase *Presence of which of the following differentiates* at the beginning of item stems. Here's a typical example:

> Presence of which of the following differentiates heart failure in hyperthyroidism from heart failure in chronic mitral regurgitation?
>
> A. Elevated systemic vascular resistance
> B. Pulmonary crackles
> C. Peripheral edema
> D. Elevated cardiac output
> E. Atrial fibrillation

This item asks you to define which condition is present *only* in heart failure associated with hyperthyroidism. Your analysis, then, might flow something like this:

- Elevated systemic vascular resistance is not characteristic of heart failure in hyperthyroidism and, therefore, is incorrect.
- Pulmonary crackles may be heard in both conditions (hyperthyroidism and mitral regurgitation) and does not differentiate between them. This response is therefore incorrect.
- Peripheral edema and atrial fibrillation are common in both conditions. Therefore, both C and E are incorrect responses.
- An elevated cardiac output is found only in hyperthyroid heart failure and, thus, D is the correct response.

Tip #3: Management Distractors

Many test items deal with the initial management of a disease or disorder. These items may contain responses beginning with *Consultation with,* followed by a physician-specialist, such as vascular surgeon, gastroenterologist, or dermatologist. Be careful of these items; there are many conditions in which the initial management involves first a medication, and *then* a consultation. Here's an example:

> A 65-year-old man has the sudden onset of a painful, cold left arm. Examination shows the left arm to be pale, cold, and numb. No brachial, radial, or ulnar pulses are felt in the affected arm. Electrocardiography shows atrial fibrillation. Which of the following is the preferred initial management?
>
> A. Administration of oral aspirin
> B. Administration of intravenous heparin
> C. Application of warm compresses to the left arm
> D. Consultation with a vascular surgeon
> E. Administration of phentolamine into the brachial artery

This patient has suffered an embolus to the brachial artery related to his atrial fibrillation. Consultation with a vascular surgeon is indicated, but consultation is not the initial step in management. Initial management involves administration of intravenous heparin prior to arrival of the surgeon.

Tip #4: Infectious Diseases

The NCCPA Content Blueprint is divided into body system categories including Infectious Diseases. Although roughly 3 percent of test items are considered part of the Infectious Diseases category, there will be many items that could fit that category. For instance, a question on acute pyelonephritis is considered by the Blueprint to be a genitourinary item, not an infectious disease item. A question on viral hepatitis is considered to be a gastrointestinal item, not an infectious disease item. And so on.

According to the Blueprint, Infectious Disease test items deal only with infectious diseases that don't have a primary target organ. Those diseases include HIV infection, AIDS, and infectious mononucleosis.

Tip #5: Assume Nothing

Experienced item writers do not use trick questions. Their items are specifically designed to find out what you know. They don't "hide" critical information, so test takers shouldn't assume that they do. Many test takers, for instance, erroneously assume that a patient has a particular disorder when in fact the test item stem indicates no such disorder. Here's an example:

> A 66-year-old man has angina pectoris associated with ventricular premature beats. Vital signs are normal. Heart and lung examination is normal. Which of the following is the preferred therapy?

This test item is trying to determine whether the test taker knows that beta-adrenergic blockers are preferred when a patient has myocardial ischemia associated with ventricular ectopy. If the test taker mistakenly assumes that the patient has insulin-dependent diabetes mellitus, he or she might answer that a calcium channel blocker is preferred.

The lesson: Do not make assumptions.

Table of Contents

Foreword vii

Preface xv

Preparing for the Exam xvii

Part I Essentials: Your Medical Information Base		1
Section 1	Essentials Review	3
Section 2	Essentials Answers	45
Part II Performance: Gauging Your Test Success		143
Section 1	Performance Test	145
Section 2	Performance Test Answers	217

Appendix: How You Can Use the NCCPA Content Blueprint to Improve Your Test Performance 241

Index 253

Part One

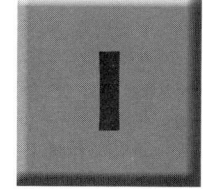

Essentials: Your Medical Information Base

ESSENTIALS is the resource that is carefully designed to enhance your clinical skills in the most important aspects of disease:

- Symptoms and signs
- Pathophysiology
- Pharmacology
- Anatomy
- Laboratory/imaging diagnostic studies
- Clinical therapeutics

ESSENTIALS is composed of didactic questions, nearly all with clinical vignettes, that will strengthen your medical information base. The questions are constructed to enable you to *compare and contrast* medical data. Therefore, many questions in **ESSENTIALS** have **more than one correct answer.** Your skill in critical thinking will be improved.

An answer section immediately follows the **ESSENTIALS** questions and contains a succinct exposition entitled **"You Should Know."**

ESSENTIALS is the medical information bridge to **PERFORMANCE.**

Section One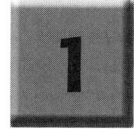

Essentials Review

Remember: There may be more than one correct answer to a question.

Organ Classification System

Although the questions are presented in random order to simulate the actual structure of the PANCE and PANRE examinations, each question has a tag identifying the organ system or systems to which that question relates. For example, a question on endocarditis will be tagged for both Infectious Disease (ID) and Cardiovascular (CV); a question on melasma will be tagged Reproductive (REPRO) and Dermatology (DERM). In this way, you may self-assess your knowledge in each of the following categories.

Cardiovascular	CV
Pulmonary	PUL
Endocrine	ENDO
Eye, Ears, Nose, and Throat	EENT
Gastrointestinal/Nutritional	GI/N
Genitourinary	GU
Musculoskeletal	MS
Reproductive	REPRO
Neurologic	NEURO
Psychiatric/Legal and Ethics	PSY/LE
Dermatologic	DERM
Hematologic/Oncology	HEME/ONC
Infectious Disease	ID

CV

E 001 Diastolic heart failure is associated with which of the following?
   A. Increased afterload
   B. Left ventricular hypertrophy
   C. Decreased left ventricular ejection fraction
   D. Systemic hypotension
   E. Mitral valve regurgitation

NEURO, PSY/LE, GI/N

E 002 Which of the following is a cause of dementia?
   A. Alzheimer's disease
   B. Folic acid deficiency
   C. Chronic alcohol abuse
   D. Parkinson's disease
   E. Huntington's chorea

PSY/LE, ENDO, HEME, NEURO

E 003 Which of the following is a cause of *reversible* dementia?
   A. Hypothyroidism
   B. Depression
   C. Pernicious anemia
   D. Bismuth poisoning
   E. Normal pressure hydrocephalus

GI/N, HEME

E 004 Which of the following conditions may cause jaundice?
   A. Hemolysis
   B. Pancreatic carcinoma
   C. Acute viral hepatitis
   D. Gilbert's disease
   E. Pulmonary infarction

GI/N, HEME

E 005 Which of the following conditions is associated with an increase in serum unconjugated ("indirect") bilirubin?
   A. Hemolysis
   B. Physiologic jaundice in the newborn
   C. Gilbert's disease
   D. Dubin-Johnson syndrome
   E. Metastatic tumor in the liver

HEME, GI/N

E 006 Which of the following conditions is associated with an increase in serum conjugated ("direct") bilirubin?
   A. Dubin-Johnson syndrome
   B. Biliary tract obstruction
   C. Intrahepatic cholestasis
   D. Glucose-6 phosphate dehydrogenase deficiency
   E. Metastatic tumor in the liver

CV

E 007 Which of the following may cause a patient to have myocardial ischemia?

   A. Atherosclerosis
   B. Coronary artery spasm
   C. Left ventricular hypertrophy
   D. Anomalous coronary artery
   E. Infiltrative myocardial disease

DERM, GI/N, NEURO

E. 008 Which of the following is a side effect of niacin therapy?

   A. Flushing
   B. Pruritus
   C. Nausea
   D. Paresthesias
   E. Peripheral edema

CV

E 009 Which of the following is a cardiovascular complication of cocaine use?

   A. Acute myocardial infarction
   B. Dissection of the aorta
   C. Ventricular tachycardia
   D. 1st degree atrioventricular block
   E. Myocarditis

GI/N, MS

E 010 Which of the following is an extra-intestinal manifestation of Crohn's disease (regional enteritis)?

   A. Arthritis
   B. Cholelithiasis
   C. Cerebral berry aneurysm
   D. Clubbing
   E. Pulmonary fibrosis

HEME

E 011 Which of the following laboratory values would be expected in a patient who has hemolysis?

   A. Decreased serum haptoglobin
   B. Increased serum lactic dehydrogenase
   C. Increased reticulocyte percentage
   D. Decreased serum gamma-glutamyl transpeptidase
   E. Decreased serum ferritin

GI/N, NEURO

E 012 Which of the following is a complication of cirrhosis of the liver?

A. Esophageal varices
B. Spontaneous bacterial peritonitis
C. Encephalopathy
D. Hepatocellular carcinoma
E. Spontaneous arterial thrombosis

CV

E 013 Which of the following medications slows atrioventricular conduction?

A. Digoxin
B. Metoprolol
C. Nifedipine
D. Captopril
E. Diltiazem

CV, GU

E 014 Which of the following conditions is associated with increased central venous pressure?

A. Superior vena cava syndrome
B. Right heart failure
C. Constrictive pericarditis
D. Nephrotic syndrome
E. Cirrhosis

CV

E 015 Which of the following is the preferred initial test to confirm the diagnosis of an acute thoracic dissection of the aorta?

A. Chest radiograph
B. Magnetic resonance imaging (MRI) of the thorax
C. Transesophageal echocardiogram
D. Computed tomography (CT) of the thorax
E. Contrast aortography

DERM, HEME, GI/N

E 016 Which of the following may cause pruritus?

A. Polycythemia rubra vera
B. Primary biliary cirrhosis
C. Nonsteroidal anti-inflammatory medications
D. Legionnaires' disease
E. Renal cell carcinoma

CV, GU, ENDO

E 017 In which of the following diseases is angiotensin-converting enzyme inhibitor therapy indicated?

A. Diabetic nephropathy
B. Systolic heart failure
C. Acute interstitial nephritis
D. Primary hyperaldosteronism
E. Pheochromocytoma

CV, GU

E 018 Which of the following conditions is associated with acute pericarditis?

A. Isoniazid hydrazide therapy
B. Systemic lupus erythematosus
C. Uremia
D. Angiotensin-converting enzyme inhibitor therapy
E. Levodopa therapy

CV, ENDO

E 019 Which of the following is a cause of orthostatic hypotension?

A. Chronic adrenal insufficiency
B. Diabetic autonomic insufficiency
C. Hypovolemia due to blood loss
D. Pheochromocytoma
E. Subclavian steal syndrome

GI/N, MS

E 020 Which of the following medications causes painful swallowing due to esophagitis?

A. Doxazosin
B. Amoxicillin
C. Sumatriptan
D. Digoxin
E. Alendronate

NEURO

E 021 Which of the following is associated with an intention tremor?

A. Myasthenia gravis
B. Parkinson's disease
C. Amyotrophic lateral sclerosis
D. Cerebellar degeneration
E. Multiple sclerosis

CV

E 022 An increased serum level of C-reactive protein is associated with increased risk of which of the following?

A. Acute myocardial infarction
B. Venous thromboembolism
C. Rheumatoid arthritis
D. Carcinoma of the colon
E. Glaucoma

CV, NEURO

E 023 Which of the following is characteristic of a vasovagal reaction?

A. Palpitations
B. Cold sweat
C. Headache
D. Wheezing
E. Diarrhea

NEURO, CV

E 024 Which of the following may cause syncope in an 80-year-old man?

A. Acute myocardial infarction
B. Sick sinus syndrome
C. Orthostatic hypotension
D. Acute mesenteric ischemia
E. Subarachnoid hemorrhage

PUL, CV

E 025 Which of the following is a typical clinical finding in the patient who has chronic bronchitis complicated by right heart failure?

A. Systemic arterial hypoxemia
B. Pulmonary hypertension
C. Anemia
D. Leucocytosis
E. Peripheral edema

PSY/LE, NEURO, ENDO

E 026 Which of the following is a side effect of lithium therapy?

A. Tremor
B. Hypothyroidism
C. Cogwheel rigidity
D. Diarrhea
E. Hyperchloremic acidosis

NEURO

E 027 Which of the following is a clinical symptom associated with atherosclerotic stenosis of a carotid artery?

A. Vertigo
B. Urinary incontinence
C. Transient visual loss in one eye
D. Fatigue
E. Transient difficulty in speaking

PSY/LE

E 028 Which of the following is a characteristic of attention-deficit hyperactivity disorder?

A. Impulsivity
B. Inattention
C. Urinary incontinence
D. Association with congenital heart anomalies
E. Association with other psychiatric conditions

DERM, PUL

E 029 Which of the following is a common food allergen in a 3-year-old child?

A. Wheat
B. Eggs
C. Milk
D. Oats
E. Beef

GI/N

E 030 Which of the following is the pathophysiologic abnormality in infants who have Hirschsprung's disease?

A. Deficiency of bile salts in the ileum
B. Absence of ganglion cells in the colon
C. Presence of an abnormal transmitter at neuromuscular junctions
D. Presence of autoimmune receptor blockers in colonic mucosa
E. Hypersecretion of Brunner's glands in the duodenum

ENDO

E 031 Which of the following medicines may cause hyperglycemia?

A. Prednisone
B. Niacin
C. Naproxen
D. Pravastatin
E. Diltiazem

DERM, ENDO, GI/N

E 032 Which of the following conditions is associated with acanthosis nigricans?

A. Obesity
B. Diabetes mellitus
C. Gastrointestinal cancer
D. Cushing's syndrome
E. Systemic lupus erythematosus

GU, GI/N, ENDO

E 033 Which of the following is a cause of hypokalemia?

A. Diarrhea
B. Primary hyperaldosteronism
C. Furosemide therapy
D. Aspirin poisoning
E. Acute renal failure

GU, PUL

E 034 Which of the following is a therapeutic intervention in the treatment of hyperkalemia?

A. Intravenous calcium
B. Intravenous sodium bicarbonate
C. Hemodialysis
D. Intravenous hypertonic saline
E. Inhaled albuterol

ID, NEURO, HEME, CV

E 035 Which of the following is a complication of infectious mononucleosis?

A. Aseptic meningitis
B. Bell's palsy
C. Hemolytic anemia
D. Pericarditis
E. Nephrotic syndrome

EENT

E 036 Which of the following is a complication of contact lens?

A. Acanthamoeba keratitis
B. Chalazion
C. Blepharitis
D. Corneal ulceration
E. Keratoconjunctivitis sicca

NEURO, EENT

E 037 Which of the following is a maneuver that tests function of cranial nerve VII?

A. Move eyes in vertical gaze
B. Frown
C. Curl tongue
D. Raise shoulders against resistance
E. Rapid repetition of a three-word phrase

HEME, GU

E 038 Which of the following serum laboratory values is typically elevated in the tumor lysis syndrome?

A. Potassium
B. Sodium
C. Uric acid
D. Norepinephrine
E. 5-hydroxy indole acetic acid

PUL, GU

E 039 An increased serum level of which of the following is consistent with a diagnosis of sarcoidosis?

A. Calcium
B. Immunoglobulin A
C. Anti-phospholipid antibodies
D. Angiotensin-converting enzyme
E. Creatine kinase

EENT, NEURO

E 040 Which of the following diseases is a cause of diplopia?

A. Cranial nerve III palsy
B. Myasthenia gravis
C. Bell's palsy
D Multiple sclerosis
E. Trigeminal neuralgia

NEURO, CV, GU

E 041 Which of the following congenital disorders is associated with cerebral aneurysm?

A. Coarctation of the aorta
B. Polycystic kidney disease
C. Tetralogy of Fallot
D. Congenital adrenal hyperplasia
E. Ostium primum atrial septal defect

CV

E 042 Which of the following is a complication of acute dissection of the thoracic aorta?

A. Pericardial tamponade
B. Left pleural effusion
C. Aortic valve regurgitation
D. Acute myocardial infarction
E. Papillary muscle rupture

GI/N, REPRO, CV

E 043 Which of the following must be considered in a patient who is to start tetracycline therapy?

   A. Ingestion of milk
   B. Concomitant intake of warfarin
   C. Concomitant intake of oral contraceptives
   D. Ingestion of aluminum-containing antacids
   E. Concomitant intake of digoxin

GI/N

E 044 Which of the following suggests an esophageal motility disorder as the etiology of dysphagia?

   A. Presence of anemia
   B. Dysphagia in conjunction with heartburn
   C. Occurrence of hematemesis
   D. Dysphagia to solids and liquids at onset of symptoms
   E. Dysphagia to liquids prior to solids

CV

E 045 In a patient who has an acute myocardial infarction complicated by pulmonary edema, which of the following medications is contraindicated?

   A. Streptokinase
   B. Nitroglycerin
   C. Aspirin
   D. Metoprolol
   E. Heparin

CV

E 046 In a patient who has an acute myocardial infarction complicated by hypertension and pulmonary edema, which of the following medications is the preferred therapy?

   A. Intravenous nitroglycerin
   B. Intravenous diazoxide
   C. Intravenous labetalol
   D. Sublingual captopril
   E. Oral ingestion of liquid nifedipine

CV, GU

E 047 Which of the following increases the risk of toxicity in a patient taking digoxin?

   A. Hypomagnesemia
   B. Hypokalemia
   C. Iron deficiency anemia
   D. Hypo-osmolar serum
   E. Hypernatremia

Section 1 ■ **Essentials Review** 13

CV, NEURO

E 048   Which of the following is an indication for verapamil therapy?
        A. Variant angina pectoris
        B. Migraine headaches
        C. Ventricular ectopic beats
        D. Hypertension
        E. Hypertrophic obstructive cardiomyopathy

GU, HEME

E 049   Which of the following conditions is associated with hematuria?
        A. Acute glomerulonephritis
        B. Renal cell carcinoma
        C. Cystitis
        D. Henoch-Schönlein purpura
        E. Polycystic kidney disease

HEME, GI/N, ENDO

E 050   Which of the following is a cause of macrocytosis?
        A. Alcohol ingestion
        B. Liver disease
        C. Hypothyroidism
        D. Chronic adrenal insufficiency
        E. Bronchiectasis

HEME, GI/N,

E 051   Which of the following is a cause of vitamin B_{12} deficiency?
        A. Pernicious anemia
        B. Strict vegan diet
        C. Crohn's disease
        D. Hypertriglyceridemia
        E. Sulfonylurea medication

NEURO, ENDO

E 052   Which of the following diseases is associated with antibody formation?
        A. Myasthenia gravis
        B. Graves' disease
        C. Hashimoto's disease
        D. Systemic lupus erythematosus
        E. Sarcoidosis

EENT

E 053 Eosinophiles are found in the nasal secretions in which of the following disorders?

A. Allergic rhinitis
B. Nasal polyposis
C. Viral rhinitis
D. Rhinitis medicamentosa
E. Bacterial sinusitis

CV

E 054 Which of the following medications may cause orthostatic hypotension?

A. Hydralazine
B. Isosorbide dinitrate
C. Niacin
D. Risperidone
E. Diltiazem

HEME, ID

E 055 In which of the following diseases are petechiae typically found on physical examination?

A. Aplastic anemia
B. Meningococcemia
C. Endocarditis
D. Rocky Mountain spotted fever
E. Polycythemia rubra vera

EENT, PUL

E 056 Which of the following disorders may be complicated by the development of nasal polyps?

A. Chronic allergic rhinitis
B. Cystic fibrosis
C. Bronchiectasis
D. Rhinitis medicamentosa
E. Vasomotor rhinitis

CV, ENDO

E 057 In a patient with newly diagnosed hypertension, which of the following suggests a secondary cause of the elevated blood pressure?

A. Radial-femoral arterial pulse lag
B. Rounded face and buffalo hump
C. Orthostatic hypotension
D. Acanthosis nigricans
E. Spooning of fingernails

PUL, CV

E 058 Which of the following disorders is associated with clubbing of the fingers and toes?

A. Chronic obstructive pulmonary disease
B. Metastatic cancer in the lung
C. Cyanotic congenital heart disease
D. Endocarditis
E. Cystic fibrosis

CV, ENDO

E 059 Which of the following is associated with an increased pulse pressure on physical examination?

A. Increasing age
B. Hyperthyroidism
C. Aortic valve regurgitation
D. Cushing's syndrome
E. Pulmonic stenosis

NEURO, HEME

E 060 On physical examination, which of the following neurologic signs is abnormal in a patient who has pernicious anemia?

A. Stereognosis
B. Extraocular muscle movements
C. Vibratory sensation
D. Proprioception
E. Romberg test

NEURO, ID, ENDO

E 061 Which of the following disorders may cause cranial nerve palsy?

A. Lyme disease
B. Cerebral aneurysm
C. Sarcoidosis
D. Diabetes mellitus
E. Myasthenia gravis

ENDO, PSY/LE, CV

E 062 Which of the following medications may cause the patient to become hypothyroid?

A. Radioactive iodine
B. Amiodarone
C. Lithium
D. Cholestyramine
E. Furosemide

GI/N, HEME, NEURO

E 063 Which of the following is a consequence of chronic alcohol abuse?

  A. Hypomagnesemia
  B. Folic acid deficiency
  C. Wernicke's encephalopathy
  D. Adenomatous polyps of the colon
  E. Hypertrophic cardiomyopathy

CV

E 064 A child with congenital long QT interval is most likely to faint during which of the following activities?

  A. Straining at stool
  B. Arising quickly from bed
  C. Gulping a very cold drink
  D. Vomiting
  E. Playing volleyball

ENDO, DERM, CV, GI/N

E 065 Which of the following is associated with chronic primary adrenal insufficiency (Addison's disease)?

  A. Weight loss
  B. Nausea
  C. Hyperpigmentation of the skin
  D. Orthostatic dizziness
  E. Weakness

MS

E 066 A 70-year-old man has diffuse bone pain. Evaluation confirms the diagnosis of Paget's disease of bone. Which abnormal laboratory value is expected in this patient?

  A. Hypercalcemia
  B. Increased serum alkaline phosphatase level
  C. Increased serum gamma-glutamyl transpeptidase level
  D. Increased urinary hydroxyproline level
  E. Increased hemoglobin level

CV

E 067 Which of the following medicines may cause peripheral edema?

  A. Diltiazem
  B. Ibuprofen
  C. Captopril
  D. Doxazosin
  E. Aspirin

ID, CV

E 068 A 72-year-old man has chronic stable angina pectoris. He received his only pneumococcal vaccination at age 69 years. Which of the following is the recommendation for this patient?

A. Revaccination at age 74 years
B. No need for revaccination
C. Revaccination only if patient develops pneumococcal pneumonia
D. Revaccination only if patient moves to adult congregate facility
E. Revaccination based upon antibody titer to *Streptococcus pneumoniae*

CV, PUL

E 069 A 79-year-old woman has a 1-week history of worsening dyspnea. She has smoked cigarettes for many years and has a history of remote myocardial infarction. Which of the following blood diagnostic studies is most appropriate to determine the cause of the dyspnea?

A. Nt-BNP (brain natriuretic peptide)
B. Troponins
C. C-reactive protein
D. Systemic arterial pO2 (PaO_2)
E. Alpha-1 anti-trypsin

CV

E 070 Which of the following is the recommended medicine to initiate therapy in an adult hypertensive patient who is otherwise well?

A. Angiotensin-receptor blocker
B. Angiotensin-converting enzyme inhibitor
C. Thiazide
D. Alpha-adrenergic blocker
E. Calcium channel blocker

GU, CV

E 071 Which of the following medicines is contraindicated in the man who takes sildenafil?

A. Isosorbide dinitrate
B. Doxazosin
C. Adenosine
D. Captopril
E. Verapamil

DERM

E 072 Which of the following skin disorders may have pustular lesions?

A. Rosacea
B. Tinea barbae
C. Impetigo
D. Lichen planus
E. Scabies

CV, PUL

E 073 Which of the following is the primary pathophysiologic abnormality in cor pulmonale?

  A. Decreased right ventricular afterload
  B. Increased left atrial pressure
  C. Hypercarbia
  D. Respiratory alkalosis
  E. Pulmonary hypertension

PSY/LE

E 074 Which of the following psychotropic medicines may cause an extrapyramidal adverse effect?

  A. Haloperidol (Haldol)
  B. Thiothixene (Navane)
  C. Fluphenazine (Prolixin)
  D. Diazepam
  E. Sertraline (Zoloft)

CV, GI/N, GU

E 075 Which of the following is a potential adverse effect of nonaspirin, nonselective, nonsteroidal anti-inflammatory medicines (NSAIDs)?

  A. Heart failure
  B. Peptic ulcer
  C. Azotemia
  D. Hypernatremia
  E. Increased anion gap metabolic acidosis

HEME, GI/N

E 076 A patient who takes methotrexate for treatment of malignant disease should be advised to do which of the following?

  A. Take daily supplement of colchicine
  B. Take daily supplement of folic acid
  C. Drink 24 ounces of milk daily
  D. Avoid intake of raw vegetables
  E. Take daily supplement of omega-3 fish oil

GI/N, PUL

E 077 The risk of acetaminophen toxicity is increased in the patient who is characterized by which of the following?

  A. Has chronic alcohol abuse
  B. Takes cyclophosphamide (Cytoxan)
  C. Takes isoniazid
  D. Takes captopril
  E. Is older than 80 years of age

MS

E 078 After an evening of excessive beer intake, a 59-year-old man suddenly awakens with severe pain at the base of the left great toe. The joint is swollen and exquisitely tender. Which of the following is the preferred initial therapy?

A. Aspirin
B. Acetaminophen
C. Indomethacin
D. Probenecid
E. Allopurinol

CV, ID

E 079 A 50-year-old man has a mechanical prosthetic heart valve. Endocarditis prophylaxis is recommended if the patient is to undergo which of the following procedures?

A. Dental extraction
B. Transurethral resection of the prostate
C. Endoscopic retrograde cholangiography
D. Percutaneous balloon angioplasty
E. Endodontic root canal

ID

E 080 A 17-year-old woman has a 2-day history of fever, sore throat, myalgia, and fatigue. Exam shows diffuse, symmetrical lymphadenopathy, inflamed tonsils with exudates, and palatal petechiae. Which of the following is the most likely diagnosis?

A. Hodgkin's disease
B. Infectious mononucleosis
C. Sarcoidosis
D. Tonsillar abscess
E. Angioneurotic edema

DERM

E 081 Which of the following is characterized by annular lesions?

A. Psoriasis
B. Secondary syphilis
C. Tinea versicolor
D. Tinea corporis
E. Henoch-Schönlein purpura

DERM

E 082 A 26-year-old man has pruritic lesions on his elbows, knees, and glans penis. There are annular red plaques with silvery scales. No lymphadenopathy is noted. The palms are not affected. Which of the following is the most likely diagnosis?

A. Psoriasis
B. Secondary syphilis
C. Drug eruption
D. Erythema migrans
E. Kaposi sarcoma

I/N, ID, REPRO, GU

E 083 Which of the following is associated with an elevated serum amylase level?

A. Acute pancreatitis
B. Mumps
C. Mesenteric infarction
D. Ruptured ectopic pregnancy
E. Renal failure

GI/N

E 084 An 83-year-old man with chronic systolic heart failure has a blood urea nitrogen (BUN) value of 41 mg/dL and a serum creatinine of 1.4 mg/dL. Which of the following is the most likely cause of the elevated BUN/creatinine ratio?

A. Acute tubular necrosis
B. Bilateral ureteral obstruction
C. Renal hypoperfusion
D. Decreased muscle mass
E. Iron deficiency anemia

ENDO

E 085 In addition to a deficiency in islet cell response to glucagon, which of the following is the pathophysiologic abnormality in type 2 diabetes mellitus?

A. Tissue resistance to insulin
B. Increased hepatic gluconeogenesis
C. Deficient level of glucose-6 phosphate dehydrogenase
D. Autoimmune destruction of B pancreatic cells
E. Defect in oxidative metabolism

CV, ENDO, REPRO

E 086 A 32-year-old obese, sedentary woman has hypertension, fasting plasma triglyceride of 400 mg/dL, serum uric acid of 8.1 mg/dL, and fasting plasma glucose of 114 mg/dL. Her menstrual cycles are regular. Examination shows normal hair distribution. Which of the following is the most likely diagnosis?

A. Cushing syndrome
B. Metabolic syndrome
C. Polycystic ovary syndrome
D. Resorptive hypercalciuria
E. Type 2 diabetes mellitus

CV, MS

E 087 In a patient who has new-onset hypertension, verapamil is preferred therapy over hydrochlorothiazide in a patient who has which of the following?

A. Claudication of the legs
B. Gout
C. Chronic obstructive lung disease
D. Tachy-brady syndrome (sick sinus)
E. Cholelithiasis

PUL

E 088 Several days after an upper respiratory infection, a healthy 4-year-old girl has community acquired pneumonia. Which of the following is the most likely infecting organism?

A. Respiratory syncytial virus
B. *Streptococcus pneumoniae*
C. *Chlamydia pneumoniae*
D. Hantavirus
E. Varicella

GI/N

E 089 Which of the following is a risk factor for gastric adenocarcinoma?

A. *Helicobacter pylori* gastritis
B. Pernicious anemia
C. Candidal esophagitis
D. Gastroesophageal reflux
E. Billroth I gastroduodenostomy

ID

E 090 Which of the following is considered to be a high-risk infectious disease from a bioterrorist attack?

A. Plague
B. Lassa fever
C. Tularemia
D. Dengue fever
E. Anthrax

CV, GU

E 091 A 42-year-old woman is transported to the emergency department after having suffered extensive hemorrhaging in a vehicular accident. Blood pressure is 70/40 mm Hg; pulse, 140/min; and respirations, 29/min. Infusion of which of the following is the preferred initial therapy?

A. Normal saline
B. Half-normal saline
C. Dextrose 5% in water
D. Dextrose 5% in half-normal saline
E. Dextrose 5% with dopamine

CV

E 092 A 66-year-old man has acute, severe hypovolemia. Which of the following is an expected sign?

A. Elevated central venous pressure
B. Orthostatic hypotension
C. Loud first heart sound (S1)
D. Warm, moist skin
E. Flushing

PSY/LE

E 093 A patient is diagnosed as having panic disorder. Which of the following is a clinical manifestation of this condition?

A. Panic episodes are typically unrelated to menses
B. Tends to be familial
C. Increased risk of suicide
D. Onset usually under age 25 years
E. Increased association with obsessive-compulsive disorder

GI/N, REPRO, CV

E 094 Which of the following is associated with ascites formation?

A. Cirrhosis
B. Left heart failure
C. Peritoneal carcinomatosis
D. Cholecystitis
E. Polycystic ovary syndrome

ENDO, GI/N

E 095 Which of the following suggests that a diabetic patient has developed gastroparesis?

A. Poor glycemic control despite vigorous measures
B. Nocturnal wheezing attacks
C. Hematemesis
D. Vomiting of bile-stained material
E. Residual food in stomach after overnight fast

CV, HEME

E 096 Which of the following is the pathophysiologic mechanism by which cyclo-oxygenase 2 (COX 2) inhibitors increase the risk of arterial thrombosis?

A. Increased effect of prostacyclin
B. Increased marrow production of platelets
C. Increased presence of Factor V Leiden
D. Production of anti-phospholipid antibodies
E. Unopposed effect of thromboxane

CV, NEURO

E 097 Which of the following is an absolute contraindication to thrombolytic therapy?

A. Active internal bleeding
B. Blood pressure 230/120 mm Hg
C. Trauma causing syncope within 4 weeks
D. Previous hemorrhagic stroke
E. Intracranial neoplasm

DERM

E 098 Which of the following is characteristic of uncomplicated herpes zoster infection?

A. Pain may precede rash
B. Rash is unilateral
C. Rash is macular eruption
D. Only occurs in immunocompromised persons
E. Rash occurs along course of a nerve

MS, ID

E 099 An increased risk for which of the following is the basis for not recommending fluoroquinolones to a patient who is under 18 years of age?

A. Uveitis
B. Erosion of joint cartilage
C. Allergic pneumonitis
D. Chemical hepatitis
E. Aseptic necrosis

ENDO, GI/N

E 100 A 57-year-old man follows a Mediterranean diet. Which of the following is an expected result?

A. Reduced low-density lipoprotein (LDL) cholesterol
B. Reduced insulin resistance
C. Reduced C-reactive protein
D. Increased platelet agglutination
E. Reduced prostaglandin activity

PUL

E 101 A 62-year-old woman has a nonproductive cough for the past 2 weeks. Which of the following medicines may be the causative factor?

A. Diltiazem
B. Doxazosin
C. Hydrochlorothiazide
D. Clonidine
E. Captopril

PUL, ID

E 102 The primary goal of Pneumonia Patient Outcomes Research Team (PORT) is which of the following?

A. Define specific antibiotic for treatment of pneumonia
B. Select patients requiring intensive care unit
C. Identify patients requiring pneumococcal vaccine
D. Select low-risk patients for outpatient treatment
E. Identify patients requiring intubation

CV, ENDO, GU, REPRO

E 103 A patient who has which of the following diseases should be treated with an angiotensin-converting enzyme inhibitor (ACEI)?

A. Acute anterior wall myocardial infarction
B. Diabetic nephropathy
C. Hypertensive diabetic without nephropathy
D. Amyloidosis
E. Hypertensive heart disease

PUL

E 104 A 64-year-old man with a long history of smoking has a 3-month history of progressive weakness and increasing cough. In the past week, he has twice coughed up a teaspoonful of red blood. Examination shows a wasted man with a firm right supraclavicular node, decreased tactile fremitus, and absent breath sounds over the lower half of the right posterior chest. Which of the following is the most likely diagnosis?

A. Squamous cell carcinoma of lung with effusion
B. Adenocarcinoma of lung with effusion
C. Atelectasis
D. Bronchiectasis
E. Right pneumothorax

PUL

E 105 A 54-year-old woman is receiving heparin for treatment of deep vein thrombosis. A normal value of which of the following is considered to be most specific in excluding a complicating pulmonary embolism?

A. Serum brain natriuretic peptide
B. Systemic arterial pCO2 (Pa_{CO_2})
C. Serum D-dimer
D. Systemic arterial pO2 (Pa_{O_2})
E. Right ventricular chamber volume on echocardiography

MS, ENDO

E 106 Three days after hitting her right calf against a coffee table, a 57-year-old diabetic woman has aching pain in the affected calf. Examination shows erythema and a palpable linear venous cord in the right calf. No edema is present. Which of the following is the most likely diagnosis?
   A. Superficial phlebitis
   B. Deep vein thrombosis
   C. Cellulitis
   D. Erythema nodosum
   E. Necrobiosis lipoidica diabeticorum

CV, ENDO, MS

E 107 Which of the following may be associated with high cardiac output heart failure?
   A. Arteriovenous fistula
   B. Hyperthyroidism
   C. Paget's disease of bone
   D. Beriberi
   E. Aortic valve regurgitation

GU, CV, ENDO, GI/N

E 108 In a patient who has metabolic acidosis, which of the following is the most important laboratory determination to be made?
   A. Osmolal gap
   B. Auscultatory gap
   C. Systemic arterial carboxyhemoglobin
   D. Anion gap
   E. Left ventricular end-diastolic pressure

MS, REPRO, ENDO

E 109 Which of the following conditions may be complicated by carpal tunnel syndrome affecting both hands and wrists?
   A. Acromegaly
   B. Hypothyroidism
   C. Rheumatoid arthritis
   D. Amyloidosis
   E. Pregnancy

ID, REPRO, ENDO

E 110 In which of the following patients is live attenuated influenza vaccine recommended?
   A. Chronic obstructive lung disease
   B. Diabetes mellitus
   C. 48-year-old healthy woman
   D. Pregnant woman
   E. Person with egg allergy

ENDO, CV, EENT, REPRO

E 111 A 41-year-old woman has a 3-week history of insomnia, increased warmth, tremulousness, and palpitations. Blood pressure is 160/60 mm Hg; pulse, 122/min; and respirations, 19/min. Examination shows lid lag and exophthalmos. Which of the following is the most likely diagnosis?

   A. Toxic adenoma of the thyroid
   B. Factitious hyperthyroidism
   C. Graves' disease
   D. Thyrotropin-secreting pituitary tumor
   E. Thyroiditis

NEUR, ID

E 112 Suspicion of which of the following is an indication for performing lumbar puncture?

   A. Meningitis
   B. Subarachnoid hemorrhage
   C. Multiple sclerosis
   D. Guillain-Barré syndrome
   E. Lewy body dementia

ID, GI/N

E 113 Which of the following is an organism that causes an infectious, noninflammatory diarrhea?

   A. Norovirus
   B. Rotavirus
   C. Enterotoxigenic *Escherichia coli*
   D. *Staphylococcus aureus*
   E. *Giardia*

GI/N

E 114 Which of the following is a typical manifestation of ulcerative colitis?

   A. Bloody diarrhea
   B. Abscess formation
   C. Fecal urgency
   D. Megaloblastic anemia
   E. Malabsorption syndrome

GI/N, EENT, PUL

E 115 Which of the following is a symptom that may be related to gastroesophageal reflux?

   A. Hoarseness
   B. Wheezing
   C. Water brash
   D. Diarrhea
   E. Loss of taste

PUL, CV

E 116 A 67-year-old man is receiving external radiation therapy for squamous cell carcinoma of the lung. He now has a 2-day history of aching discomfort in the left calf with associated edema in the affected calf and left ankle. The calf discomfort increases with walking, particularly when ascending stairs. Examination shows mild erythema and edema of the left calf and ankle. The affected calf is warm. No inguinal lymph nodes are felt. Which of the following is the most likely diagnosis?

A. Metastatic carcinoma to left tibia
B. Superficial phlebitis
C. Deep vein thrombosis
D. Paraneoplastic syndrome
E. Cellulitis

CV

E 117 A 43-year-old obese man has 30 minutes of diffuse anterior chest pain that is associated with sweating. Vital signs are normal. The patient is not cyanotic. Lungs are clear to auscultation. Heart tones are distant, but no murmur, gallop, or friction rub is heard. No peripheral edema is present. Homans' sign is negative. The patient's electrocardiogram is shown. Which of the following is the most likely diagnosis?

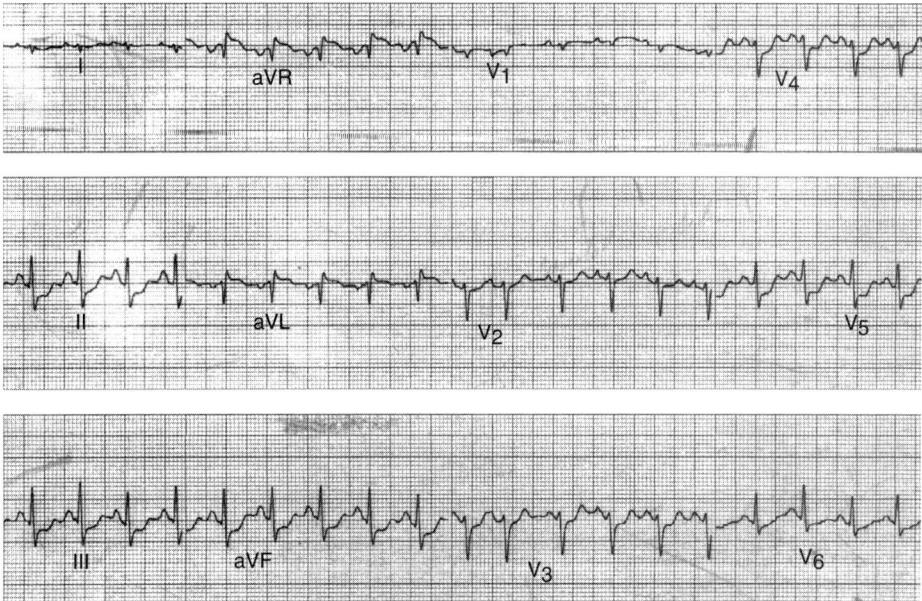

A. Acute pericarditis
B. Pleurodynia
C. Dissection of the aorta
D. Acute coronary syndrome
E. Acute pulmonary embolism

REPRO

E 118   Which of the following is a risk factor for a pregnant woman to develop preeclampsia?

   A. Cigarette smoking
   B. Past history of preeclampsia
   C. Family history of preeclampsia
   D. First pregnancy
   E. Anti-phospholipid antibodies

REPRO

E 119   Seven weeks after her last menstrual period, a 32-year-old woman has amenorrhea, abdominal pain, and vaginal bleeding. In addition to serum human chorionic gonadotropin concentration, which of the following is the preferred test to diagnose ectopic pregnancy?

   A. MRI scan of the pelvis
   B. Culdocentesis
   C. Curettage
   D. Serum progesterone level
   E. Transvaginal ultrasonography

ID, GI/N

E 120   A 34-year-old man has the following hepatitis B serologic markers: HBsAg positive; IgM-anti-HBc positive. Which of the following is the most likely status of the patient?

   A. Susceptible to hepatitis B infection
   B. Immune to natural infection
   C. Immune due to hepatitis B immunization
   D. Chronic hepatitis B infection
   E. Acute hepatitis B infection

REPRO

E 121   Which of the following is considered to be the least important indication for cesarean delivery?

   A. Failure to progress in labor
   B. Fetal distress
   C. Previous cesarean delivery
   D. Breech lie
   E. Under 1500 g birth weight baby

GI/N

E 122   A 49-year-old man has acute, severe, right upper quadrant abdominal pain, fever with chills, and jaundice. Blood pressure is 106/72 mm Hg; pulse, 120/min; and axillary temperature 102°F. White blood cell count is 29,200/µL; hemoglobin, 13.1 g/dL. Which of the following is the preferred initial diagnostic test?

   A. Transhepatic cholangiogram
   B. Endoscopic retrograde cholangiography
   C. Hepatic iminodiacetic acid (HIDA) scan
   D. Intravenous cholangiogram
   E. Percutaneous liver biopsy

GU/REPRO

E 123 Which of the following is the primary pathophysiological mechanism that is associated with primary dysmenorrhea?

A. Impaired release of nitric oxide from arcuate arteries
B. Decreased estrogen stimulation of the endometrium
C. Heightened progestin stimulation of the endometrium
D. Increased secretion of luteinizing hormone
E. Prostaglandin induction of uterine contraction

PSY/LE, GU

E 124 A 32-year-old woman has premenstrual dysmorphic disorder. Her usual activity is impaired by which of the following?

A. Bloating
B. Hopelessness
C. Anger
D. Peripheral edema
E. Mood lability

GI/N, ID

E 125 A 36-year-old man has active upper gastrointestinal bleeding requiring transfusion. Which of the following is the preferred diagnostic test for diagnosis of *Helicobacter pylori* infection?

A. Fecal antigen immunoassay
B. Gastric biopsy
C. ELISA serology
D. Blood culture
E. Urea breath test

GI/N, ID

E 126 Active *Helicobacter pylori* gastritis is diagnosed in a 51-year-old woman who has recurrent epigastric pain. Which of the following agents is not used in therapy?

A. Clarithromycin
B. Amoxicillin
C. Bismuth subsalicylate
D. Metronidazole
E. Ceftriaxone

ENDO, CV, GU

E 127 A 27-year-old man is in diabetic ketoacidosis. Blood pressure is 72/58 mm Hg; pulse, 146/min; respiratory rate, 36/min. Examination shows dry oral mucosa and poor turgor. Plasma glucose is 642 mg/dL; serum potassium, 3.2 mEq/L; and systemic arterial pH, 6.8. Which of the following is the preferred initial intravenous solution to be infused?

A. 0.9% saline
B. 0.45% saline
C. Ringer's lactate
D. 2 ½% dextrose in normal saline
E. 3% saline

ENDO

E 128 A 52-year-old obese man has newly diagnosed type 2 diabetes mellitus. Which of the following is the preferred initial therapy?

- A. Metformin
- B. Rosiglitazone
- C. Miglitol
- D. Nateglinide
- E. Glipizide

ID, PUL

E 129 In the midst of a recognized influenza outbreak, a 34-year-old woman has fever, chills, sore throat, muscle aching, and cough productive of mucoid sputum. Which of the following should not be prescribed?

- A. Ibuprofen
- B. Oseltamivir
- C. Acetaminophen
- D. Iodopropylidine glycerol
- E. Amantadine

GU

E 130 Which of the following conditions is associated with hypokalemia?

- A. Pheochromocytoma
- B. Loop diuretic therapy
- C. Lidocaine therapy
- D. Angiotensin-converting enzyme inhibitor therapy
- E. Alkalosis

NEURO

E 131 Antibodies to acetylcholine receptors are typically found in a patient who has which of the following conditions?

- A. Myasthenia gravis
- B. Multiple sclerosis
- C. Amyotrophic lateral sclerosis
- D. Guillain-Barré syndrome
- E. Hashimoto's disease

GU, CV

E 132 A 62-year-old man has diabetic nephropathy with nephrotic syndrome. Which of the following is least likely to be noted in the patient?

- A. Hyperlipidemia
- B. Hypercoagulable state
- C. Hypoalbuminemia
- D. Oral fat bodies in the urine
- E. Hypertension

HEME, CV

E 133 A 56-year-old man has a 2-week history of night sweats. Which of the following may be the underlying etiology?

A. Cushing's disease
B. Endocarditis
C. *Helicobacter pylori* gastric ulcer
D. Sarcoidosis
E. Lymphoma

NEURO

E 134 Which of the following is the pathophysiologic abnormality in the brain that results in primary parkinsonism?

A. Dopamine depletion
B. Serotonin depletion
C. Increased activity of the reticulostriate system
D. Decreased parasympathetic tone
E. Increased neuronal uptake of norepinephrine

GI/N, ID

E 135 A 74-year-old man undergoes a partial gastrectomy for carcinoma of the stomach. Three hours after surgery, after the patient has been extubated, the patient's rectal temperature is 100.8°F. Vital signs are normal. Lungs are clear to auscultation. A Foley catheter is anchored. Arterial blood gas values are normal. Which of the following is the most likely cause of the fever?

A. Atelectasis
B. Urinary tract infection
C. Surgical wound infection
D. Tissue release of cytokines
E. Aspiration pneumonia

NEURO, CV

E 136 A 78-year-old man is diagnosed as having subclavian steal syndrome. Which of the following symptoms are consistent with this diagnosis?

A. Monocular blurred vision
B. Arm claudication
C. Dizziness
D. Diplopia
E. Binocular blurred vision

GU

E 137 A 26-year-old black man who suffers from heroin addiction acutely develops nephrotic syndrome. Which of the following is the most likely diagnosis?

A. Amyloidosis
B. Systemic lupus erythematosus
C. Multiple myeloma
D. Fibrillary glomeruloscleronephritis
E. Focal glomerulosclerosis

REPRO

E 138 Which of the following is a risk factor for sudden infant death syndrome (SIDS)?

A. Maternal smoking during pregnancy
B. Low birth weight infant
C. Prone sleeping position
D. Maternal history of diabetes mellitus
E. Patent foramen ovale in the infant

REPRO, GU

E 139 Which of the following is an absolute contraindication to the use of oral contraceptives?

A. Diabetes mellitus
B. Benign tumor of the liver
C. History of spontaneous abortion
D. Chronic glomerulonephritis
E. Migraine

ENDO, CV

E 140 A 62-year-old woman takes glyburide for type 2 diabetes mellitus. Additional therapy with which of the following medicines is most likely to facilitate the onset of hypoglycemia?

A. Propranolol
B. Indomethacin
C. Diltiazem
D. Chlorpromazine
E. Levodopa

ENDO, REPRO

E 141 A 24-year-old healthy primigravida of Native American ancestry should have plasma glucose determination after a 50 g oral glucose load at which of the following times during the pregnancy?

A. Between 16 and 20 weeks
B. Between 30 and 36 weeks
C. As soon as pregnancy is determined
D. Between 24 and 28 weeks
E. Only if ketonuria is present

REPRO, CV

E 142 In the 23rd week of gestation, a previously normotensive 27-year-old primigravida has serial blood pressure determinations averaging 142/94 mm Hg. There is no proteinuria. In addition to restricted activity, which of the following is preferred management?

A. Initiate therapy with oral methyldopa
B. No medicinal therapy at this time
C. Initiate therapy with oral hydralazine
D. Initiate therapy with oral labetalol
E. Initiate therapy with sublingual nifedipine

HEME, GI/N

E 143 Which of the following is a cause of iron deficiency?

A. Intravascular hemolysis
B. Celiac disease
C. *Helicobacter pylori* gastritis
D. Carcinoma of the cecum
E. Graves' disease

NEURO, GU

E 144 Serum alpha-fetoprotein levels are used to screen for which of the following conditions?

A. Neural tube defects
B. Tetralogy of Fallot
C. Wilms' tumor of the kidney
D. Hepatic vein thrombosis
E. Germ cell tumor of the testis

GU, HEME

E 145 A dipstick urinalysis in a 44-year-old man is positive for blood. Microscopic examination of the urine reveals no red blood cells. Presence of which of the following in the urine is most likely?

A. Myoglobin
B. Hemosiderin
C. Phenazopyridine (Pyridium)
D. Waxy casts
E. Immunoglobulins

ID, DERM, EENT

E 146 A 12-year-old boy has a 5-day history of fever, headache, and rhinorrhea after which a rash appears. Examination shows a bilateral erythematous malar rash with circumoral pallor. Which of the following organisms is the most likely cause of the illness?

A. Adenovirus
B. *Streptococcus pyogenes*
C. Coxsackievirus
D. Parvovirus
E. Herpes simplex 1 virus

ID

E 147 Which of the following is the pathophysiologic abnormality that is primarily responsible for opportunistic infection in the AIDS patient?

A. Hypercatabolism of immunoglobulin proteins
B. Decreased serum complement (C3) concentration
C. Impaired opsonization
D. Impaired cellular immunity
E. Immunoglobulin loss in urine

ID

E 148 A 36-year-old man with AIDS has a CD4 cell count of <50 cells/μL. Tuberculin skin test shows 6 mm induration. He should not receive prophylaxis against which of the following infections?

A. *Mycobacterium avium* complex
B. Toxoplasmosis
C. *Pneumocystis carinii*
D. *Candida*
E. Tuberculosis

NEURO, EENT, ENDO

E 149 After 4 days of aching discomfort in the right eye, a 52-year-old diabetic man has diplopia. Examination shows ptosis of the right eyelid and the right eye is in a position of abduction. The pupils are normal in size and equal. Which of the following is the most likely diagnosis?

A. Subarachnoid hemorrhage
B. Lyme disease
C. Cranial nerve V mononeuropathy
D. Cervical spondylosis
E. Cranial nerve III mononeuropathy

NEURO, ENDO, GU, CV

E 150 Which of the following is a manifestation of diabetic autonomic neuropathy?

A. Gastroparesis
B. Orthostatic hypotension
C. Nocturnal diarrhea
D. Retrograde ejaculation
E. Brady-tachy syndrome

REPRO

E 151 At 31 weeks of gestation, a 32-year-old G4 P2 woman has the sudden onset of profuse, painless vaginal bleeding. Which of the following is the most likely diagnosis?

A. Abruptio placentae
B. Threatened abortion
C. Ectopic pregnancy
D. Placenta previa
E. Hydatidiform mole

HEME

E 152 A 34-year-old woman is to undergo elective splenectomy for hereditary spherocytosis. Administration of which of the following is recommended prior to the surgery?

A. Oral folinic acid
B. Intravenous immunoglobulin
C. Oral metronidazole
D. *Haemophilus influenzae* conjugate vaccine
E. Platelet transfusion

GI/N

E 153 A 47-year-old man has alcoholic cirrhosis with ascites. Which of the following is a precipitating cause of hepatic encephalopathy?

A. Hypovolemia
B. Hypokalemia
C. Gastrointestinal bleeding
D. Spironolactone therapy
E. Administration of a lactulose enema

GU, ENDO, HEME

E 154 A 67-year-old man with type 1 diabetes mellitus has end-stage renal disease. Which of the following is an expected laboratory abnormality to be noted in this patient?

A. Hypokalemia
B. Hypercalcemia
C. Hyperphosphatemia
D. Macrocytic, nonmegaloblastic anemia
E. Normocytic normochromic anemia

GU, CV

E 155 A 78-year-old man has chronic systolic heart failure with a left ventricular ejection fraction of 24%. Therapy includes a loop diuretic, beta-adrenergic blocker, and angiotensin-converting enzyme inhibitor. The heart failure is most likely to be associated with which of the following?

A. Metabolic acidosis
B. Hyperchloremia
C. Hyperkalemia
D. Elevated serum osmolality
E. Hyponatremia

CV, GU

E 156 Which of the following conditions may precipitate generalized seizures?

A. Hyponatremia
B. Hypocalcemia
C. Transient ischemic attack
D. Uremia
E. Encephalitis

GU

E 157 Over a period of 3 days, an 87-year-old man who is bedridden has worsening mental status and then becomes delirious. Serum sodium is 156 mEq/L. Which of the following is the most likely cause?

A. Hepatic encephalopathy
B. Hyperglycemia
C. Acute adrenal insufficiency
D. Hypertriglyceridemia
E. Dehydration

ENDO

E 158 Which of the following may be a clinical manifestation of hypoglycemia?

A. Sweating
B. Confusion
C. Seizures
D. Thirst
E. Polyuria

ID, GU

E 159 Infection with human papillomavirus may cause which of the following conditions?

A. Carcinoma of the cervix
B. Chancroid
C. Granuloma inguinale
D. Condylomata acuminata
E. Plantar warts

NEURO, GI/N

E 160 Forty-eight hours after his last drink, a 67-year-old man with chronic alcohol abuse has hallucinations, disorientation, and agitation. Examination shows a confused patient with profuse diaphoresis, low-grade fever, and tachycardia. Which of the following is the most likely diagnosis?

A. Delirium tremens
B. Alcoholic hallucinosis
C. Pheochromocytoma
D. Malignant neuroleptic syndrome
E. Korsakoff's syndrome

GI/N

E 161 A 3-week-old infant male has immediate postprandial, nonbilious vomiting. Examination shows a small rounded mass at the lateral edge of the rectus abdominis muscle in the right upper quadrant. Which of the following is the most likely diagnosis?

A. Hypertrophic pyloric stenosis
B. Intussusception
C. Hirschsprung's disease
D. Congenital diaphragmatic hernia
E. Umbilical hernia

ENDO

E 162 A 66-year-old woman has type 2 diabetes mellitus. Metformin therapy has resulted in fasting plasma glucose levels in the 160 to 170 mg/dL range. Blood urea nitrogen, serum creatinine, and liver function values are normal. Which of the following is the preferred additional therapy?

A. NPH insulin
B. Acarbose
C. Glipizide
D. Nateglinide
E. Rosiglitazone

PSY/LE

E 163 During a commercial airline flight the captain requests assistance from an onboard passenger who is a medical professional. Under which of the following conditions does the Samaritan lose legal protection under the Aviation Medical Assistance Act of 1998?

A. Fails to hold current professional licensure
B. Fails to obtain sick passenger's consent
C. Fails to produce written documentation of intervention
D. Fails to directly communicate with captain
E. Receives monetary compensation

HEME, ID

E 164 Intravenous immune globulin is administered to a patient who has which of the following conditions?

A. Multiple myeloma
B. Multiple sclerosis
C. Polyarteritis nodosa
D. Idiopathic thrombocytopenic purpura
E. Kawasaki disease

GI/N

E 165 Presence of which of the following differentiates chronic liver failure from the previously healthy patient who now has acute, fulminant liver failure?

A. Jaundice
B. Spider angiomata
C. Ascites
D. Asterixis
E. Encephalopathy

REPRO, GI/N, CV

E 166 Which of the following is an absolute contraindication to oral contraceptive therapy?

A. Hypertriglyceridemia
B. Chronic active hepatitis
C. History of deep vein thrombosis
D. 1st degree relative with ovarian cancer
E. Atrial fibrillation

ENDO

E 167 Which of the following is associated with hyperglycemia?

A. Polycystic ovary syndrome
B. Hypercortisolism
C. Acromegaly
D. Pheochromocytoma
E. Medullary carcinoma of the thyroid

GU, CV

E 168 Which of the following medicines may cause hypertension?

A. Lithium
B. Doxazosin
C. Fluoxetine
D. Naproxen
E. Sildenafil

ID, HEME

E 169 Which of the following diseases is associated with eosinophilia?

A. Trichinellosis
B. Ascariasis
C. Systemic lupus erythematosus
D. Multiple sclerosis
E. Meningococcemia

CV

E 170 Which of the following is a risk factor for dissection of the aorta?

A. Hypertension
B. Muscular dystrophy
C. Use of crack cocaine
D. Tetralogy of Fallot
E. Marfan's syndrome

NEURO, EENT

E 171 Presence of which of the following differentiates vertigo related to brainstem disease ("central" vertigo) from vertigo related to inner ear disease ("peripheral" vertigo)?

A. Dysmetria
B. Nystagmus
C. Head extension exacerbates vertigo
D. Association with herpes zoster
E. Tinnitus

NEURO, HEME

E 172 A 22-year-old man who lives in a residence with a poorly functioning heating system has a severe headache and mild confusion. Which of the following is the preferred diagnostic test for carbon monoxide poisoning?

A. Pulse oximetry
B. Systemic arterial pO2 (PaO_2)
C. Venous cyanhemoglobin
D. Systemic arterial methemoglobin
E. Systemic arterial carboxyhemoglobin

Section 1 ▪ Essentials Review

GU

E 173 Presence of which of the following clinical signs differentiates torsion of the appendix testis from testicular torsion?

A. Fever and chills
B. Urethral discharge
C. Long axis of testis is oriented horizontally
D. Abdominal wall reflexes
E. Cremasteric reflex

NEURO

E 174 A 52-year-old man has a 3-hour history of diffuse headache. Presence of which of the following historical factors is suggestive of a life-threatening headache?

A. Sudden onset
B. Association with nasal congestion
C. Association with tearing
D. Pulsating quality
E. Onset with physical exertion

GU, ID

E 175 A 27-year-old healthy, nonpregnant woman has a 2-day history of dysuria and urinary frequency without fever. Microscopic analysis of a clean-catch urine specimen shows pyuria and bacteriuria. Which of the following is the most appropriate management?

A. 1 day of nitrofurantoin therapy
B. 3 days of fluoroquinolone therapy
C. 1 day of trimethoprim-sulfamethoxazole therapy
D. 7 days of ampicillin therapy
E. 7 days of tetracycline therapy

ID, GU

E 176 A 32-year-old man has a 2-day history of fever, dysuria, urinary frequency, and perineal discomfort. Examination shows a tender, swollen prostate. Which of the following is the most likely infecting organism?

A. *Enterobacter* species
B. *Acinetobacter* species
C. *Moraxella catarrhalis*
D. *Proteus vulgaris*
E. *Escherichia coli*

NEURO

E 177 Which of the following is most likely to be considered a normal variant upon examination of a vigorous 81-year-old man?

A. Loss of proprioception in the toes
B. Unilateral facial anhidrosis
C. Stocking glove sensory loss in the lower legs
D. Unilateral extensor Babinski response
E. Absence of bilateral ankle deep tendon reflexes

DERM

E 178   A 46-year-old woman has a 1-week history of a rash involving her chest, scalp, and inguinal areas. The rash is depicted in the photograph. Which of the following is the most likely diagnosis?

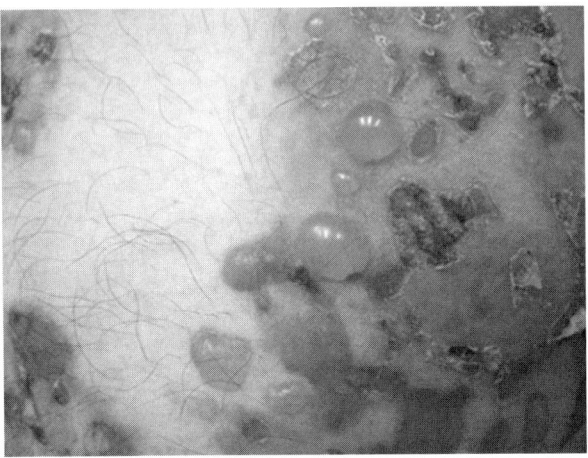

A. Lichen simplex chronicus
B. Miliaria
C. Pemphigus
D. Contact dermatitis
E. Atopic dermatitis

DERM, ID

E 179   A 52-year-old obese man has a 1 week history of burning in the groin area. The area is shown in the photograph. Which of the following is the preferred initial diagnostic test?

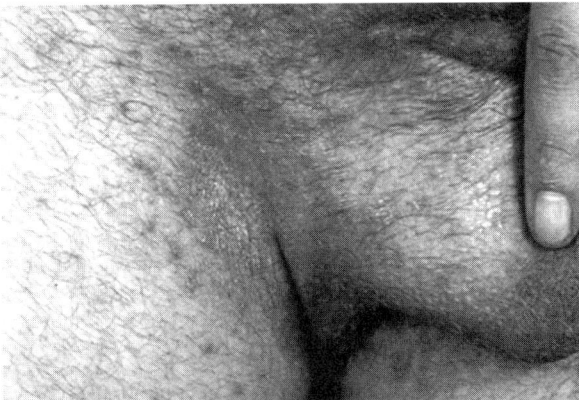

A. Potassium hydroxide preparation of rash debris
B. Bacterial culture and sensitivity of rash debris
C. Polymerase chain reaction
D. Anti-streptolysin O titer
E. Examination under Wood's lamp

CV

E 180 Upon routine examination, an asymptomatic 14-year-old boy is noted to have a heart murmur. His electrocardiogram is shown. Which of the following is the most likely diagnosis?

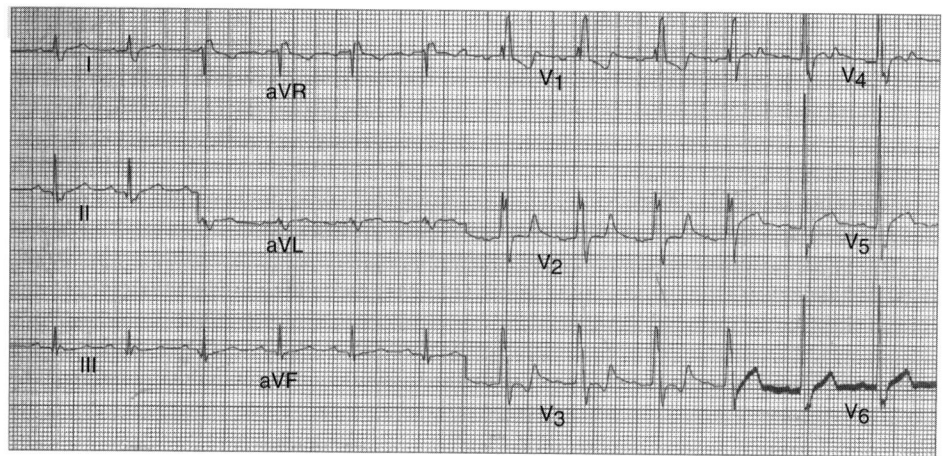

A. Atrial septal defect
B. Ventricular septal defect
C. Aortic valve stenosis
D. Tetralogy of Fallot
E. Mitral valve prolapse

CV

E 181 A 26-year-old woman has the sudden onset of palpitations described as very fast and regular. Blood pressure is 110/60 mm Hg and respiratory rate is 24/min. The patient is alert and pink. No heart murmur or gallop is heard. Chest radiography is normal. The patient's electrocardiogram is shown. Which of the following is the preferred initial therapy?

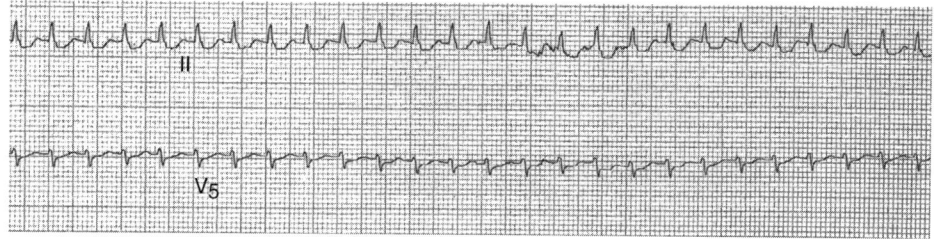

A. Intravenous lidocaine
B. Oral verapamil
C. Sublingual nifedipine
D. Intravenous adenosine
E. Emergent cardioversion

DERM, ID

E 182   During a very hot and humid summer, a 34-year-old man has a 1-week history of a rash on his trunk. The rash does not involve the palms and soles. The rash is shown in the photograph. Which of the following is the most likely diagnosis?

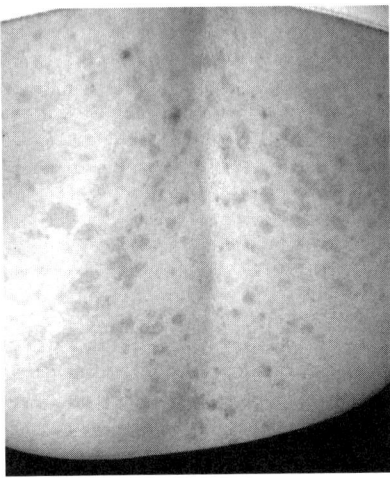

A. Secondary syphilis
B. Erythema multiforme
C. Bullous pemphigoid
D. Rocky Mountain spotted fever
E. Tinea versicolor

DERM, REPRO

E 183   A 27-year-old woman has a 1-month history of an asymptomatic rash on both cheeks. The rash is shown in the photograph. Which of the following is the most likely associated condition?

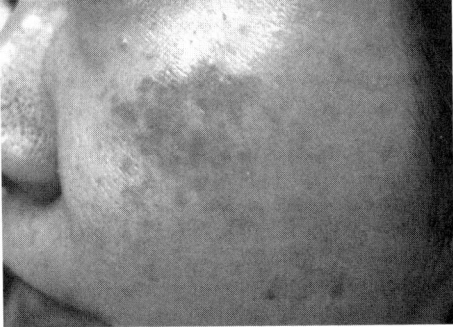

A. Cushing's disease
B. Oral intake of diltiazem
C. Oral intake of omeprazole
D. Pregnancy
E. Rheumatoid arthritis

DERM, ID

E 184 A 41-year-old man has a 2-day history of a rash that is shown in the photographs. The skin disorder is most likely to be associated with which of the following?

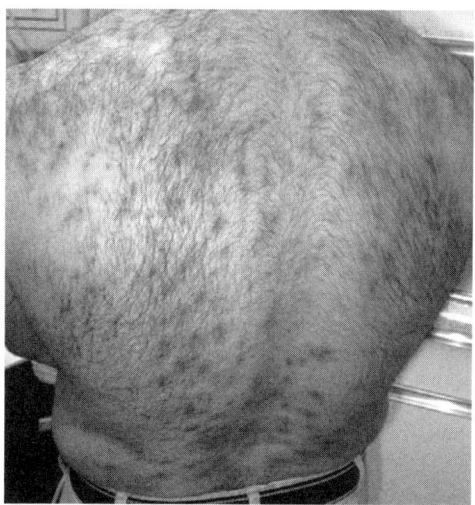

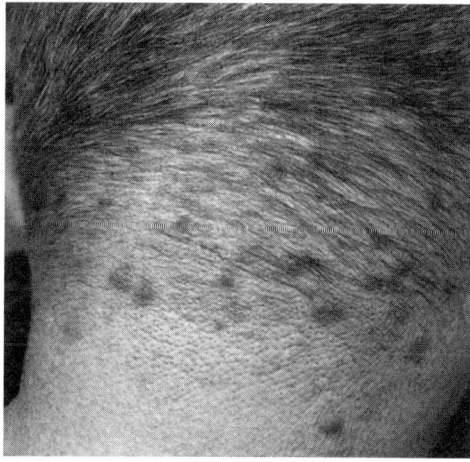

A. Bathing in a hot tub
B. Exposure to ultraviolet radiation
C. Ingestion of sulfites
D. Vitamin A poisoning
E. Adverse reaction to verapamil

ID, PUL

E 185　A healthy 34-year-old man who lives in Arizona has a 3-day history of fever, minimally productive cough, and right pleuritic chest pain. He now has erythema nodosum on the anterior surface of both lower legs. Which of the following is the preferred initial diagnostic test to confirm the diagnosis of coccidioidomycosis?

　　A. Sputum culture and sensitivity
　　B. Skin test to coccidioidomycosis antigens
　　C. Tube precipitin test
　　D. Latex test
　　E. Biopsy of erythema nodosum lesion

Photos for questions *E 178, E 179, E 182, E 183,* and *E 184* from: Barankin, B, and Freiman, A. Derm Notes: Clinical Dermatology Pocket Guide. Philadelphia: F.A. Davis Company, 2006.

Section Two

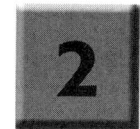

Essentials Answers

E 001 **Answer: A and B**

A and B are correct because increased afterload causes left ventricular hypertrophy (LVH). The left ventricular hypertrophy (LVH) causes the ventricle to be stiff resulting in diastolic heart failure (HF) with its associated dyspnea.

■ You Should Know

1. Diastolic heart failure is due to increased stiffness (decreased compliance) of the left ventricle (LV). In order to effectively fill the left ventricle (LV) during diastole, left atrial pressure must increase. This increased pressure is transmitted backwards to the lung. Therefore, the cardinal symptom of diastolic heart failure (HF) is *dyspnea*, treated with diuretics.

2. Diastolic heart failure (HF) is most often associated with left ventricular hypertrophy (LVH). LVH is the compensatory response to increased afterload from systemic hypertension or aortic valve stenosis. The physical sign of left ventricular hypertrophy (LVH) is an apical lift or heave, often accompanied by an S4 gallop if the patient is in sinus rhythm.

3. The left ventricular hypertrophy (LVH) may be secondary to *acquired* disease (e.g., hypertension or aortic valve stenosis) or due to *congenital* disease (e.g., hypertrophic cardiomyopathy or coarctation of the aorta).

4. Other causes of increased left ventricle (LV) stiffness include infiltrative myocardial disease (e.g., amyloidosis) and myocardial ischemia. Myocardial ischemia causes a *transient* increase in stiffness, thus explaining the brief dyspnea that often accompanies angina pectoris. "Anginal equivalent" is dyspnea (*without anginal discomfort*) of brief duration that is due to ischemia.

5. In addition to diuretics, diastolic heart failure (HF) is treated with beta-adrenergic blockers, which improve ventricular filling by slowing the heart rate, and with nondihydropyridine calcium channel blockers (verapamil and diltiazem), which improve ventricular compliance.

E 002 **Answer: A, C, D, and E**

A, C, D, and E are correct because dementia occurs in Alzheimer's disease, chronic alcohol abuse, Huntington's chorea, and Parkinson's disease.

You Should Know

1. Dementia is a syndrome characterized by deterioration of cognitive abilities manifest by memory loss and impairment in calculation, judgment, and problem solving. It is often associated with social deficits including depression, agitation, hallucinations, and insomnia.

2. Dementia due to chronic alcohol abuse is related to malnutrition, especially of the B vitamins, and particularly thiamine.

3. Dementia is six times more common in Parkinson's disease than in the general population. Treatment of Parkinson's disease with anticholinergic medications or amantadine often worsens the cognitive deficits in the patient.

4. Huntington's disease, also associated with dementia, is inherited in an autosomal dominant manner. It is associated with chorea, characterized by involuntary rapid, jerky motions.

E 003 **Answer: A, B, C, D, and E**

A, B, C, D, and E are correct because dementia may be the result of endocrine (hypothyroidism), hematologic (pernicious anemia), psychiatric (depression), and neurologic disease (normal pressure hydrocephalus). If diagnosed early and treated, the dementia is reversible. Further, bismuth poisoning is potentially reversible.

You Should Know

1. The clinician must always search for treatable (reversible) causes of depression.

2. Depression may masquerade as dementia with apparent memory loss and impaired judgment ("pseudodementia"). Treatment of the depression results in improved cognitive function.

3. Vitamin B_{12} deficiency may cause dementia while the blood elements are *completely normal* (i.e., normal hemoglobin, red blood cell indices, and number of segments in the neutrophils). The patient's dementia may make examination of the posterior spinal columns (proprioception and vibratory sensation) impossible. A serum vitamin B_{12} level should be obtained. Be aware, however, that even a normal serum vitamin B_{12} level does not completely rule out this diagnosis. Neurology consultation is advised.

4. Patients having normal pressure hydrocephalus will have dementia plus abnormal gait and urinary incontinence. Ventricular shunting surgery will improve the mental faculty in half of the operated patients.

5. Considerable intake of oral bismuth, as in treatment of *Helicobacter pylori* infection, may cause dementia, particularly in the patient who has underlying renal insufficiency.

6. Hypothyroid patients often have memory loss and depression, in addition to cold intolerance, weight gain, and weakness. Serum thyroid-stimulating hormone (TSH) is elevated in primary hypothyroidism and normal or low in secondary hypothyroidism.

E 004 **Answer: A, B, C, and D**

A, B, C, and D are correct because jaundice may be due to hematologic disease (hemolysis) or hepatobiliary disease (intrahepatic or extrahepatic obstruction to bilirubin excretion).

■ **You Should Know**

1. Jaundice may be due to *either* increased unconjugated ("indirect") or increased conjugated ("direct") serum bilirubin levels.

2. Carcinoma of the pancreas causes jaundice when it obstructs the biliary tree.

3. Viral hepatitis produces jaundice in the obstructive phase of the illness.

4. Gilbert's disease, an inherited disorder of the liver, causes jaundice due to accumulation of indirect (unconjugated) bilirubin in the serum.

E 005 **Answer: A, B, and C**

A is correct because both extravascular hemolysis and intravascular hemolysis result in increased levels of serum unconjugated bilirubin. B is correct because physiologic jaundice in the newborn is unconjugated hyperbilirubinemia due to increased bilirubin production and decreased bilirubin clearance. C is correct because Gilbert's disease is an inherited disorder in which there is a defect in conjugation of bilirubin.

■ **You Should Know**

1. Both *extravascular* hemolysis (destruction of red blood cells in the spleen, bone marrow, and liver) and intravascular hemolysis result in increased levels of serum unconjugated bilirubin.

2. Gilbert's disease is more common in males. Other routine laboratory tests in the patient are usually normal. Prognosis appears to be the same as the general population.

E 006 **Answer: A, B, C, and E**

A is correct because Dubin-Johnson is a hereditary disorder in which there is an elevation in serum conjugated bilirubin. B, C, and E are correct because in intrahepatic cholestasis, biliary tract obstruction and metastatic tumor in the liver, the hepatocytes are able to conjugate the bilirubin, but not to normally remove it in the biliary system. Therefore, conjugated bilirubin spills from the hepatocytes into the serum causing jaundice from conjugated hyperbilirubinemia.

■ **You Should Know**

1. G-6 PD deficiency is an X-linked disorder in which patients may have acute hemolysis related to infections, medications, or stress. In these patients, hemolysis would cause an increase in unconjugated serum bilirubin.

2. Dubin-Johnson syndrome is an inherited disorder in which the patient has mild icterus but is usually otherwise asymptomatic. While the serum direct bilirubin level is elevated, the remainder of liver function tests, namely, prothrombin time, aminotransferases, and alkaline phosphatase, are normal.

E 007   Answer: A, B, C, and D
A is correct because atherosclerotic narrowing of a coronary artery causes myocardial ischemia when myocardial oxygen demand exceeds oxygen delivery through the stenotic artery (e.g., with physical effort or emotional distress). B is correct because coronary artery spasm can provoke ischemia without increased oxygen demand on the heart. C is correct because left ventricular hypertrophy (LVH) can cause myocardial ischemia in the absence of coexistent atherosclerosis or coronary spasm. D is correct because infants born with an anomalous coronary artery (e.g., the right coronary artery arising from a pulmonary artery) have myocardial ischemia starting at birth.

■ You Should Know

1. Spasm is the mechanism in variant angina (Prinzmetal's angina), a condition more common in women and causing anginal discomfort (with associated electrocardiographic ST segment *elevation*) during the very early morning hours. This is treated with calcium channel blockers and nitrates.

2. Left ventricular hypertrophy may be secondary to acquired disease (e.g., aortic valve stenosis), or due to congenital disease (e.g., hypertrophic cardiomyopathy).

3. Children with an anomalous coronary artery may begin to experience angina pectoris during childhood or young adult years. Remember: children may have angina pectoris!

4. In contrast to the electrocardiographic abnormality in variant angina, the classic electrocardiographic expression of myocardial ischemia is horizontal ST segment depression.

E 008   Answer: A, B, C, and D
A, B, C, and D are correct because flushing is the most common side effect, affecting approximately 75% of patients; pruritus, paresthesias, and nausea affect approximately 20%.

■ You Should Know

1. Niacin reduces serum cholesterol, LDL cholesterol, VLDL, and triglycerides. It increases serum high-density lipoprotein (HDL) cholesterol levels.

2. The onset of hepatotoxicity is not predictable; therefore, serial monitoring of liver function tests is essential.

3. Short-acting niacin preparations appear to have less hepatotoxicity than long-acting preparations.

4. Other side-effects include hyperglycemia and elevation of serum uric acid. Niacin should not be given to a patient who has a history of gout.

E 009   Answer: A, B, C, and E
A, B, C, and E are correct because cocaine causes stimulation of both alpha- and beta-adrenergic receptors. Cocaine usage results in hypertension and tachycardia, and

may provoke angina pectoris and myocardial infarction (due to coronary artery spasm), myocarditis, supraventricular and ventricular arrhythmias, and dissection of the aorta.

■ You Should Know

1. Administration of a pure beta-adrenergic blocker (e.g., propranolol) may worsen cocaine-induced hypertension. Beta blocker administration would result in unopposed alpha stimulation by the cocaine, thus resulting in higher systemic arterial pressure.

2. Treatment of myocardial ischemia/infarction secondary to cocaine includes a benzodiazepine anxiolytic agent, aspirin, nitrates, calcium blocker, and alpha-adrenergic blocker. (Some will use a combined alpha- and beta-adrenergic blocker, e.g., labetalol.)

3. Myocardial infarction is usually due to profound coronary artery spasm. Myocardial infarction most often occurs in patients with normal coronary arteries. In some cases, infarction is related to thrombus formation. Coronary angiography is often performed on an emergent basis in these patients.

4. Cardiovascular effects of ephedrine-containing substances (e.g., "herbal ecstasy") cause similar adrenergic hyperactivity.

E 010   **Answer: A, B, and D**
A is correct because Crohn's disease (and ulcerative colitis) has arthritic manifestations including large joint arthritis and spondylitis. B is correct because cholelithiasis is common in Crohn's disease due to malabsorption of bile salts from the terminal ileum. D is correct because clubbing occurs in inflammatory bowel disease.

■ You Should Know

1. Clubbing of the fingers and toes may be noted in patients with chronic lung infections, bronchiectasis, lung malignancy, cyanotic congenital heart disease, and endocarditis.

E 011   **Answer: A, B, and C**
A is correct because haptoglobin binds to the free hemoglobin that is released during hemolysis. This binding leads to a decrease in the level of circulating haptoglobin. B is correct because lactic dehydrogenase enzyme is found in erythrocytes. Therefore, hemolysis would cause release of this enzyme into the serum. C is correct because reticulocytes are relatively immature erythrocytes that are released into the circulation in response to hemolysis or blood loss.

■ You Should Know

1. Ferritin is the major iron *storage protein*. A serum level <35 ng/mL is indicative of iron deficiency.

2. The reticulocyte count is expressed as an "index," a value >2 suggests hemolysis or blood loss.

E 012 **Answer: A, B, C, and D**
A is correct because the portal hypertension associated with cirrhosis causes development of esophageal varices. B is correct because chronic liver disease increases the risk of the patient developing spontaneous bacterial peritonitis, an infection of ascites without an apparent intraabdominal source of infection. C is correct because the cirrhotic patient has impaired ability to detoxify products of intestinal origin. D is correct because cirrhotic patients have a markedly increased risk of developing hepatocellular carcinoma (HCC).

■ **You Should Know**

1. Ascites is the most common complication of portal hypertension that occurs in the cirrhosis patient.

2. Spontaneous bacterial peritonitis (SBP) is typically manifest as fever, abdominal pain, and altered mental status; however, some patients are asymptomatic. Without early treatment, mortality is high. Nearly 70% of those who have had SBP will have a recurrence; therefore, prophylactic antibiotics are indicated.

3. Variceal hemorrhage is a manifestation of portal hypertension. Intravenous octreotide is the preferred therapy of active bleeding. When hemorrhage has ceased, beta-adrenergic blocker therapy is given in an effort to prevent recurrence.

4. Although not specific, increasing levels of serum alpha-fetoprotein should raise clinical suspicion for hepatocellular carcinoma (HCC).

E 013 **Answer: A, B, and E**
A is correct because digoxin slows atrioventricular (AV) conduction via its parasympathetic effect on the atrioventricular (AV) node. B and E are correct because beta-adrenergic blockers and the nondihydropyridine calcium channel blockers verapamil and diltiazem slow conduction velocity in the atrioventricular (AV) node. Thus, these agents are used to slow the ventricular response in patients who have atrial fibrillation (AF).

■ **You Should Know**

1. Digoxin is preferred for rate slowing in those atrial fibrillation (AF) patients who are hypotensive or who are in heart failure.

2. Nifedipine, a dihydropyridine calcium blocker, does not slow atrioventricular (AV) conduction, nor does an angiotensin-converting enzyme inhibitor.

3. In the atrial fibrillation patient who has chronic obstructive lung disease or claudication secondary to peripheral arterial disease, verapamil and diltiazem are preferred treatment because beta-adrenergic blockers may worsen both the pulmonary function and the claudication symptoms.

4. Poor control of the ventricular response in the atrial fibrillation patient, with ventricular rates chronically >100/min, may lead to development of dilated cardiomyopathy and systolic heart failure.

5. In the patient who is in normal sinus rhythm, toxic doses of digoxin, beta-adrenergic blockers, verapamil, or diltiazem may cause second-degree or third-degree atrioventricular block.

E 014   **Answer: A, B, and C**
A is correct because superior vena cava (SVC) syndrome, due to obstruction in superior vena cava (SVC) flow into the right atrium, results in elevation of the central venous pressure (CVP). B and C are correct because the hemodynamic sequelae of right heart failure and constrictive pericarditis increase central venous pressure (CVP).

■ **You Should Know**

1. Superior vena cava (SVC) syndrome is manifest by facial and upper arm swelling and cyanosis. It does not cause edema of the lower extremities. The etiology of superior vena cava (SVC) syndrome most commonly is small cell carcinoma of the lung and non-Hodgkin's lymphoma. An additional important cause is thrombosis around an indwelling central venous catheter.

2. Both right heart failure and constrictive pericarditis are manifest by bilateral peripheral edema, ascites, and hepatomegaly. The most common cause of right heart failure (HF) is chronic systolic left heart failure (HF); another important etiology is pulmonary hypertension due to pulmonary arterial obstruction (pulmonary embolism) and pulmonary parenchymal disease (pulmonary fibrosis and chronic bronchitis). The most common cause of constrictive pericarditis in the United States is prior chest radiation for malignant disease.

3. Nephrotic syndrome and advanced cirrhosis of the liver both cause hypoalbuminemia, which is clinically manifest as ascites and bilateral peripheral edema; however, it is important to note that, in these patients, the central venous pressure is normal.

E 015   **Answer: B, C, and D**
B, C, and D are correct because transesophageal echocardiography (TEE), computed tomography (CT) scan, and magnetic resonance imaging (MRI) of the thorax are all considered to be valuable in diagnosis of dissection and are considered by different medical authorities to be the preferred initial diagnostic test.

■ **You Should Know**

1. Transthoracic ultrasound and chest radiography have a lower sensitivity.

2. Aortography is not considered to be the initial diagnostic test.

E 016   **Answer: A, B, and C**
A is correct because polycythemia rubra vera often causes the patient to experience itching after a warm shower or bath. B is correct because primary biliary cirrhosis, occurring in middle-aged women, often has itching as the initial symptom. C is correct because nonsteroidal anti-inflammatory medications (NSAIDs) may cause itching without a rash.

■ **You Should Know**

1. Polycythemia rubra vera is characterized by increased hematocrit, increased white blood cell count, and variably increased platelet count, The treatment of choice is phlebotomy.

2. In primary biliary cirrhosis the serum alkaline phosphatase is elevated. Antimitochondrial antibodies are present in the serum in 95% of patients.

3. Anti-nuclear antibodies in the serum are found in primary biliary cirrhosis, systemic lupus erythematosus, rheumatoid arthritis, Sjögren syndrome, scleroderma and polymyositis.

4. Other common adverse effects of nonsteroidal anti-inflammatory medications (NSAIDs) include elevation of blood pressure, peptic ulcer, and peripheral edema. A less frequent effect is psychosis (or other mental change), especially in the elderly patient. Remember, nonsteroidal anti-inflammatory medications (NSAIDs) have anti-platelet activity and, therefore, should be discontinued before elective surgery.

E 017 **Answer: A and B**
A is correct because angiotensin-converting enzyme inhibitors (ACEI) and angiotensin-receptor blockers both reduce intraglomerular pressure and slow progression of diabetic nephropathy to end-stage renal disease. B is correct because angiotensin-converting enzyme inhibitors (ACEI) and receptor blockers reduce afterload and, therefore, are used in systolic heart failure in an effort to improve left ventricular ejection fraction.

■ **You Should Know**

1. Primary hyperaldosteronism and pheochromocytoma are preferably treated with surgical removal of the tumors.

E 018 **Answer: A, B, and C**
A is correct because isoniazid is one of several medicines that may cause acute pericarditis. B is correct because acute pericarditis is common in systemic lupus erythematosus (SLE) and may be the presenting manifestation of the disease. C is correct because uremia is a common cause of acute pericarditis.

■ **You Should Know**

1. Isoniazid, procainamide, phenytoin, hydralazine, and the penicillins may cause acute pericarditis.

2. Anemia, leucopenia, and thrombocytopenia are common hematologic abnormalities in the systemic lupus erythematosus (SLE) patient.

3. Pericardial tamponade is a fairly common complication of uremia-induced pericarditis. Dialysis is an effective modality in therapy of uremia-associated pericarditis.

E 019 **Answer: A, B, C, and D**
A is correct because chronic adrenal insufficiency causes orthostatic hypotension due to mineralocorticoid deficiency associated with the disease. B is correct because patients with diabetes mellitus often have an autonomic neuropathy that results in orthostatic hypotension. C is correct because hypovolemia from blood loss may be associated with orthostatic hypotension. D is correct because pheochromocytoma

causes hypertension, but in contrast to other hypertensive disorders, is often associated with orthostatic hypotension.

■ You Should Know

1. Hypovolemia of any etiology, including chronic adrenal insufficiency (Addison's disease) due to mineralocorticoid deficiency, blood loss, and excessive diuresis, may cause orthostatic hypotension. In these patients, the decrease in blood pressure with assumption of the standing position is associated with a compensatory increase in heart rate.

2. Addison's disease patients commonly have hyperpigmentation of the skin. Hyponatremia is noted in 90% and hyperkalemia in 65% of cases. The cosyntropin stimulation test is performed for diagnosis.

3. Diabetic autonomic insufficiency is a common cause of orthostatic hypotension. In contrast to hypovolemia, the orthostatic decrease in blood pressure is not associated with a compensatory increase in heart rate.

4. Always check sitting blood pressure and heart rate followed by standing blood pressure and heart rate in a patient who has orthostatic hypotension. The heart rate response differentiates hypovolemia from autonomic (sympathetic) insufficiency.

5. Hypovolemia causes immediate orthostatic hypotension. In contrast, the orthostatic hypotension associated with autonomic neuropathy may be manifest only after 3 to 4 minutes of standing.

E 020   **Answer: E**
E is correct because alendronate, used in the treatment of osteoporosis, is a fairly common cause of retrosternal pain and painful swallowing due to medication-induced esophagitis.

■ You Should Know

1. Patients starting alendronate should be advised to take the pill with at least 8 ounces of water and to stand or sit upright at least 30 minutes after ingestion.

E 021   **Answer: D**
D is correct because cerebellar disease causes an intention tremor, usually in conjunction with other neurologic defects, including nystagmus, ataxia, and dysmetria.

■ You Should Know

1. Familial (essential) tremor, often with an autosomal dominant inheritance character, is an intention and postural tremor, the latter signifying tremor when an extremity is outstretched (e.g., holding a glass with an extended arm). Neurologic examination is otherwise normal. If therapy is indicated, propranolol is usually the preferred initial medication.

2. Parkinson's disease causes a resting tremor. The tremor disappears during active motion, only to reappear when the extremity is again in a position of rest.

3. Myasthenia gravis, an autoimmune disorder characterized by the presence of anti-acetylcholine receptor antibodies, causes variable weakness of skeletal muscles. Diagnosis is established by response to a short-acting anticholinesterase, e.g., edrophonium or neostigmine.

E 022 Answer: A

A is correct because C-reactive protein is a potent predictor of future coronary events, e.g., unstable angina pectoris and acute myocardial infarction.

■ You Should Know

1. In addition to being a predictor of increased risk, C-reactive protein itself is prothrombotic, thus promoting occlusive thrombosis in an artery.

2. Increased serum C-reactive protein levels in apparently healthy individuals are used to determine which patients are in need of more intensive therapy (e.g., use of statins to lower LDL cholesterol).

E 023 Answer: B

B is correct because the increased parasympathetic tone associated with a vasovagal reaction is characterized by cold sweat, nausea and, commonly, fainting.

■ You Should Know

1. A vasovagal reaction is commonly precipitated by stress, either emotional or somatic (e.g., pain). Hypotension and bradycardia are typical hemodynamic features. The initial therapy is to have the person lie flat, preferably with elevation of the legs.

2. Syncope due to cardiac arrhythmia, either bradycardia or tachyarrhythmia, often occurs without premonitory symptoms.

E 024 Answer: A, B, and C

A is correct because sudden fainting without chest pain may be a presentation of acute myocardial infarction. It is in the elderly patient that syncope is most likely to be associated with infarction. B is correct because sick sinus syndrome (brady-tachy syndrome), characterized by intermittent paroxysms of supraventricular tachycardia interspersed with periods of bradycardia (e.g., marked sinus bradycardia or sinus arrest), commonly causes syncope. C is correct because orthostatic hypotension of any etiology can provoke syncope upon assumption of the upright position. (please refer to question E 019).

■ You Should Know

1. In the patient with sick sinus syndrome the cerebral ischemia responsible for the faint may be due to either the supraventricular arrhythmia with a fast ventricular rate or, obversely, to the periods of bradycardia.

2. Any elderly patient who faints, even without associated chest pain, must be evaluated for acute myocardial infarction.

3. Syncope due to arrhythmia is often not associated with premonitory symptoms.

4. Subarachnoid hemorrhage may cause coma or impaired consciousness; this is not syncope.

E 025   **Answer: A, B, and E**
A, B, and E are correct because the chronic bronchitis patient with heart failure (the "blue bloater") has hypoxemia and elevated pulmonary artery pressure. The pulmonary hypertension leads to development of right heart failure and peripheral edema.

You Should Know

1. In contrast to patients with emphysema, patients with chronic bronchitis have greater systemic arterial *desaturation* (lower pO2 [PaO_2]) and often manifest central cyanosis. Additionally, they have pulmonary hypertension that may lead to right heart failure (cor pulmonale) manifest by peripheral edema, congestive hepatomegaly, and elevated central venous pressure.

E 026   **Answer: A, B, and C**
A is correct because lithium may cause tremor. B is correct because lithium inhibits thyroid hormone synthesis and release resulting in hypothyroidism. C is correct because cogwheel rigidity may occur with long-term lithium therapy.

You Should Know

1. The tremor associated with lithium therapy, if persistent, may be treated with propranolol.

2. Hypothyroidism is common. Thyroid function studies should be performed approximately every 3 months during therapy.

3. Thiazide diuretics, but not loop diuretics, increase serum lithium levels. Therefore, lithium dosage should be reduced in the patient taking a thiazide.

4. There is increased risk of fetal abnormalities in women taking lithium during early pregnancy. Women of child-bearing age must be informed of this risk.

5. Lithium should be taken with meals in order to lessen nausea.

E 027   **Answer: C**
C is correct because carotid atherosclerotic disease commonly causes amaurosis fugax, a transient, monocular, ipsilateral (on the same side as the carotid narrowing), visual disturbance due to retinal emboli.

You Should Know

1. Amaurosis fugax generally does not last more than 1 to 2 minutes. A patient who has amaurosis fugax should undergo a duplex ultrasound study of the carotid artery.

2. Vertebrobasilar artery insufficiency frequently is manifest by impaired speech, double vision (or blurred vision in both eyes), vertigo, ataxia, and weakness.

3. Fatigue and dysarthria (impaired speech) are not characteristic symptoms of carotid artery disease.

4. Cerebral ischemia resulting from very low cardiac output due to bradycardia (e.g., 3rd degree atrioventricular block or sinus arrest) typically causes syncope rather than localized neurologic symptoms.

5. The visual disturbance associated with migraine is *bilateral* and typically lasts longer than 1 to 2 minutes. Light flashes, sparks, and stars are common.

E 028 **Answer: A, B, and E**
A and B are correct because the central manifestations of attention-deficit-hyperactivity disorder (ADHD) are impulsivity, inattention, and hyperactivity. E is correct because attention-deficit-hyperactivity disorder (ADHD) commonly occurs in conjunction with other psychiatric disorders in a patient, including mood disorders (20%), conduct disorders (20%), oppositionally defiant disorder (40%), and Tourette's syndrome (25%).

■ **You Should Know**

1. Tourette's syndrome is characterized by tics, barking of obscenities, and, often, echolalia (repetition of words or sentences said by others). Medication, if used, most commonly is a dopamine blocker.

E 029 **Answer: A, B, and C**
A, B, and C are correct because eggs, milk, peanuts, soy, and wheat are common food allergens in young children.

■ **You Should Know**

1. In older children and adolescents, fish, shellfish, and nuts are common allergens.

2. Oats and beef are not allergens.

3. Children whose allergic response includes respiratory distress or anaphylaxis should carry injectable epinephrine.

4. The differential diagnosis of food allergy includes cystic fibrosis, celiac disease, lactase deficiency, congenital intestinal malformations, and chronic bowel infection.

E 030 **Answer: B**
B is correct because Hirschsprung's disease, due to absence of ganglion cells in the colonic mucosa, results in the affected segment being unable to relax. Therefore, functional bowel obstruction results.

■ **You Should Know**

1. Hirschsprung's disease is characterized by failure of the newborn to pass meconium, followed by abdominal distention and vomiting.

2. Suction biopsy and rectal manometry are preferable to contrast radiography (barium enema) in making the diagnosis.

3. Definitive treatment is surgical.

E 031   **Answer: A and B**
A is correct because prednisone causes hyperglycemia by increasing gluconeogenesis and by inhibiting glycogen storage. B is correct because niacin induces insulin resistance, thus resulting in hyperglycemia.

■ **You Should Know**

1. Niacin causes hyperglycemia, increases serum uric acid (even precipitating acute gout), may cause hypotension when used in conjunction with vasodilators, and may exacerbate ischemic symptoms in the patient with unstable angina pectoris.

2. Additional side effects of prednisone include osteoporosis, peptic ulcer, cataracts, and skin thinning with purpura.

3. Hypercortisolism of any etiology, including prednisone therapy, Cushing's disease, and cortisol-producing adrenal adenoma or carcinoma, can be associated with these adverse effects.

4. Prednisone-induced osteoporosis is treated with a bisphosphonate.

E 032   **Answer: A, B, C, and D**
A, B, and D are correct because the common denominator in all nonmalignancy-associated cases of acanthosis nigricans is insulin resistance. Therefore, there is an association of this skin disorder with diabetes mellitus, obesity, and Cushing's syndrome. C is correct because gastric and hepatocellular cancer (and, less frequently, lung cancer) are particularly associated with acanthosis nigricans.

■ **You Should Know**

1. Acanthosis nigricans (AN) lesions are grey-brown to black, are rough, and have prominent skin lines. They most commonly occur in the axillae, back and sides of neck, and inguinal creases.

2. Acanthosis nigricans is associated with malignant and nonmalignant conditions.

3. The classic rash associated with systemic lupus erythematosus is the "butterfly" rash in the malar area of the face.

E 033   **Answer: A, B, and C**
A is correct because diarrheal stools contain considerable potassium and bicarbonate. Therefore, hypokalemia and metabolic acidosis may result, particularly with chronic diarrhea. B is correct because primary hyperaldosteronism causes renal sodium retention in the kidney and, therefore, excessive potassium loss in the urine. C is correct because loop diuretics and thiazide diuretics increase potassium loss in the urine. Without potassium supplementation, hypokalemia may result.

You Should Know

1. In a patient who takes digoxin, hypokalemia of any etiology predisposes to digoxin toxicity. Digoxin toxicity can be manifest as:
   - Ectopy, including ventricular premature beats, ventricular tachycardia, and atrial premature beats
   - Atrioventricular block, including 1st degree, 2nd degree (Mobitz I, also called Wenckebach), and 3rd degree

2. Acute renal failure causes hyperkalemia due to the kidney's inability to excrete this electrolyte.

E 034 **Answer: A, B, C, and E**

A is correct because calcium antagonizes the electrophysiologic effects of potassium. B is correct because bicarbonate causes potassium to leave the serum and enter cells. C is correct because dialysis can rapidly remove potassium from the circulation. E is correct because $beta_2$-adrenergic agonists drive potassium from the serum into cells.

You Should Know

1. Intravenous calcium is indicated in those patients with severe hyperkalemia who have marked electrocardiographic abnormalities, including loss of P waves and widening of the QRS complex. Calcium should not be given when digoxin toxicity is suspected, because calcium can worsen the effect of the digoxin.

2. Medications given to emergently lower the serum potassium include inhaled albuterol, intravenous glucose with added insulin, and intravenous sodium bicarbonate.

3. Inhaled albuterol promotes potassium entry into cells and begins to lower serum potassium in 15 to 30 minutes. This effect lasts approximately 2 hours.

4. The combination of intravenous glucose and insulin drives potassium into the cells. The effect begins in approximately 30 to 60 minutes and lasts 4 to 6 hours.

5. Sodium bicarbonate begins to lower serum potassium in 15 to 30 minutes and its effect lasts 1 to 2 hours.

6. Sodium polystyrene sulfonate, a cation exchange resin, may be given orally or as an enema in less emergent cases. Potassium levels begin to decrease in 1 to 2 hours.

7. Hemodialysis may be employed when conservative measures are ineffective or in cases of marked tissue breakdown.

E 035 **Answer: A, B, C, and D**

A and B are correct because neurologic complications of mononucleosis include aseptic meningitis, Bell's palsy, and Guillain-Barré syndrome. C is correct because hemolytic anemia, thrombocytopenia, and neutropenia are recognized hematologic complications. D is correct because acute pericarditis is an uncommon cardiac complication.

■ You Should Know

1. Diagnosis of infectious mononucleosis is most commonly based upon presence of heterophile antibodies, including the Monospot test.

2. Atypical lymphocytes on peripheral blood smear is a very common hematologic finding, but may not be seen until the third week of illness.

E 036   **Answer: A and D**
A is correct because amebas may infect the eye, especially in patients who wear contact lens and who are not careful in cleaning and storage of the lens. D is correct because corneal ulceration is the major complication of contact lens. Soft lens appear to be the primary hazard, especially with extended wear.

■ You Should Know

1. Amebas are found in soil and in chlorinated swimming pools. Keratitis is characterized by waxing and waning ocular pain, blurred vision, and conjunctival erythema.

E 037   **Answer: B**
B is correct because cranial nerve VII (facial nerve) is a motor nerve to the face, thus being responsible for facial expressions.

■ You Should Know

1. Cranial nerve VII activation causes the patient to close the eyes, frown, wrinkle the forehead, and smile. Important: the forehead receives bilateral innervation; thus, in peripheral nerve palsy (Bell's palsy) the patient is unable to wrinkle the forehead on the affected side. In central VII nerve palsy, there is drooping of the face and inability to tightly close the eyes, but the patient can wrinkle the forehead.

2. Cranial nerve V (trigeminal) has both motor and sensory function in the face. Motor function can be tested by closing the jaw against resistance or by moving the chin from side to side.

3. Cranial nerves III, IV, and VI innervate eye muscles and are responsible for extraocular muscle movements.

4. Pupil size is related to smooth muscle function. Myasthenia gravis is an autoimmune disease that affects only skeletal muscle. Extraocular muscles are skeletal muscles. Therefore, in myasthenia gravis, abnormal extraocular muscle movements and ptosis are intermittently noted, but pupil size is always normal.

5. Cranial nerve III (oculomotor nerve) palsy causes both extraocular muscle abnormalities and a dilated pupil because this nerve carries parasympathetic nerve fibers. An important clinical point: diabetes mellitus is a common cause of cranial nerve III palsy. However, in the majority of cases, the pupil size is normal in the diabetic.

6. Lyme disease is a common cause of facial nerve paralysis, at times causing bilateral Bell's palsy. The preferred initial diagnostic study is an ELISA test. Lyme disease is typically associated with headache, arthralgia or arthritis, and erythema migrans, a flat or slightly raised red lesion.

E 038 Answer: A and C

A is correct because rapid tumor cell death leads to release of potassium from cells. C is correct because nucleic acids released from dying tumor cells are converted to uric acid, thus causing the development of hyperuricemia.

■ **You Should Know**

1. Tumor lysis syndrome (TLS) occurs in patients who have rapidly proliferating malignancies that are very sensitive to chemotherapy (e.g., acute leukemia and lymphoma).

2. Chemotherapy causes rapid tumor cell death. As a result, intracellular products spill into the blood, causing hyperkalemia, hyperphosphatemia, and hyperuricemia. Tumor lysis syndrome (TLS) may result in acute renal failure requiring hemodialysis.

3. Efforts to prevent tumor lysis syndrome (TLS) include prophylactic oral allopurinol and vigorous volume expansion.

4. Carcinoid syndrome, characterized by flushing, diarrhea, wheezing (and tricuspid or pulmonary valve disease), has increased urinary excretion of 5-hydroxy indole acetic acid (5 HIAA).

E 039 Answer: A and D

A and D are correct because serum angiotensin-converting enzyme is elevated in approximately 50% of sarcoidosis cases and elevation of serum calcium is noted in 3% to 5%.

■ **You Should Know**

1. Sarcoidosis is a disease of unknown etiology that commonly targets the lungs, skin, heart, eyes, liver, and kidney. Lymphadenopathy and parotid gland enlargement are also frequently noted.

2. Pulmonary involvement typically starts with bilateral hilar enlargement (similar to Hodgkin's disease). Later in the disease course, diffuse pulmonary fibrosis (interstitial fibrosis) causes restrictive pulmonary abnormalities to be manifest.

3. Restrictive pulmonary abnormalities include increased stiffness of the lungs, hyperventilation, and reduced oxygen diffusion across the alveolar-capillary membrane but not with outflow air obstruction.

4. As a result, the systemic arterial blood gas determination in the restrictive disease patient shows respiratory alkalosis, hypoxemia (low PaO_2) and *hypocapnia* (low $PaCO_2$).

5. Pulmonary function tests in any patient who has restrictive lung disease show reduced total lung capacity and decreased carbon monoxide (CO) diffusing capacity, but forced expiratory volume 1 sec./forced vital capacity (FEV 1 sec/FVC) ratio is normal or increased.

6. In contrast, in obstructive lung disease (e.g., asthma) there is a decreased FEV 1 sec/FVC ratio.

E 040   **Answer: A, B, and D**

A is correct because cranial nerve III palsy, which causes lateral deviation of the affected eye, results in diplopia. B is correct because myasthenia gravis causes intermittent weakness in the extraocular muscles (skeletal muscles), thus resulting in diplopia. D is correct because multiple sclerosis (MS) frequently causes diplopia due to cranial nerve VI (abducens nerve) palsy.

■ **You Should Know**

1. Diplopia may be monocular or binocular.

2. Monocular diplopia (i.e., double vision with the fellow eye covered) is not due to serious systemic disease, but rather is due to refractive error or cataract.

3. Binocular diplopia (i.e., double vision with both eyes uncovered) is due to malalignment of the two eyes.

4. Binocular diplopia, when due to inflammatory, neoplastic, metabolic, or vascular disease, typically is due to impaired function of the cranial nerves that innervate the extraocular muscles, namely, cranial nerves III, IV, and VI.

5. Cerebral aneurysms are an important cause of diplopia. Aneurysms may cause cranial nerve palsy, especially involving cranial nerve III. Any patient who develops a cranial nerve palsy should be evaluated for cerebral aneurysm.

6. Oculomotor (cranial nerve III) palsy is characterized by ptosis, lateral deviation of the eye, and dilated pupil.

7. An important exception: diabetes mellitus is a common cause of cranial nerve III palsy, but in 80% of cases the pupil size is normal.

8. Wernicke's encephalopathy, associated with chronic alcohol abuse, is typically characterized by extraocular muscle dysfunction, nystagmus, and disorientation or inattentiveness.

9. Myasthenia gravis, an autoimmune disease in which antibodies to acetylcholine (ACH) receptors are present, causes diffuse, intermittent, skeletal muscle weakness. Extraocular muscle weakness is intermittent; therefore, diplopia is intermittent. The pupil size is always normal in myasthenia, because it is smooth muscle, not skeletal muscle, that influences pupil size.

10. Multiple sclerosis commonly causes optic neuritis, an inflammatory disease of the optic nerve causing eye pain with eye movement and diminished visual acuity. The eye movement disorder in multiple sclerosis (MS) is accompanied by nystagmus.

E 041   **Answer: A and B**

A and B are correct because 10% of coarctation patients and 10% of polycystic kidney disease patients have congenital cerebral aneurysms.

■ **You Should Know**

1. Coarctation patients typically have equal and bilateral hypertension in the arms, low blood pressure in the legs, and radial-femoral arterial pulse lag. Bicuspid aortic valve is found in approximately 70% of those with coarctation.

2. Cerebral aneurysms may rupture and cause subarachnoid hemorrhage, even years after surgical correction of the coarctation or treatment of the kidney disease.

3. Polycystic kidney disease, with autosomal dominant inheritance, is characterized by hematuria (microscopic or gross), hypertension, flank pain, progressive renal failure and, often, nephrolithiasis.

E 042 **Answer: A, B, C, and D**
A is correct because the dissection may rupture into the pericardial sac causing tamponade. B is correct because the dissection may rupture into the left pleural space causing a left hemothorax. C and D are correct because the dissection may cause distortion of the proximal aorta causing occlusion of a coronary artery with resultant acute myocardial infarction or distortion of the aortic cusps causing aortic valve regurgitation.

■ **You Should Know**

1. Acute thoracic aorta dissection causes tearing or ripping pain in the chest. The pain may be located in the anterior and/or posterior chest.

2. Pericardial tamponade is characterized by hypotension, tachycardia, elevated central venous pressure, and paradoxical pulse.

3. Transesophageal echocardiography (TEE), CT scan, and MRI are valuable in the diagnosis of dissection. Transesophageal echocardiography (TEE) shows diastolic collapse of the right atrium or right ventricle.

4. In any patient who has chest pain and a new murmur of aortic valve regurgitation, aortic dissection must be the initial consideration.

5. The medical treatment of dissection includes an intravenous vasodilator (e.g., nitroprusside) to lower blood pressure in addition to a beta blocker, which decreases pulsatile flow.

6. Isolated use of a vasodilator like diazoxide or hydralazine is contraindicated because these may increase shear stress on the aorta and propagate the dissection.

7. Selected patients with dissection require emergent surgical intervention.

E 043 **Answer: A, B, C, and D**
A and D are correct because aluminum-containing antacids and milk decrease the absorption of tetracycline (TCN). B is correct because tetracycline (TCN) increases the anticoagulant effect of warfarin. C is correct because tetracycline (TCN) decreases the effect of oral contraceptives.

■ **You Should Know**

1. Tetracycline (TCN) must be taken at least 2 hours apart from ingestion of milk and aluminum-containing antacids.

2. In the woman taking an oral contraceptive an additional method of birth control (e.g., barrier method) must be used during tetracycline (TCN) therapy.

E 044 **Answer: D**

D is correct because dysphagia to both solids and liquids at the onset of symptoms suggests a motility disorder in contrast to dysphagia to solids that later involves liquids that suggests mechanical esophageal obstruction.

■ **You Should Know**

1. Stricture of the esophagus is a common complication of gastroesophageal reflux (GERD).

2. Cancer of the esophagus typically causes dysphagia in the presence of weight loss and anorexia.

3. Barrett's esophagus, another complication of gastroesophageal reflux (GERD), is characterized by a change in the microscopic appearance of the esophageal mucosa, specifically, from squamous to columnar epithelium.

4. Barrett's esophagus markedly increases the risk of esophageal carcinoma (adenocarcinoma), which is one of the most rapidly increasing malignancies in the United States.

5. Dysphagia to solids and liquids is common in scleroderma. These patients commonly have Raynaud's phenomenon. This disease involves the lungs, causing pulmonary fibrosis, pulmonary hypertension, and right heart failure; heart, causing myocardial fibrosis and acute pericarditis; kidneys, causing proteinuria, renal insufficiency, and hypertension.

6. Scleroderma patients produce a number of autoantibodies, most commonly anti-nuclear antibodies (90%). There is no autoantibody that is specific for scleroderma.

E 045 **Answer: D**

D is correct because beta-adrenergic blockers are contraindicated in acute heart failure because they have a negative inotropic effect.

■ **You Should Know**

1. Beta-adrenergic blockers are indicated in chronic systolic heart failure.

2. When given to the patient with chronic systolic heart failure, the beta blockers are part of polypharmacy therapy, including nitrates, angiotensin-converting enzyme inhibitors (or receptor blockers), diuretics and, occasionally, digoxin.

E 046 **Answer: A**

A is correct because intravenous nitroglycerin lowers blood pressure (decreasing afterload) and causes venodilation (reducing preload), both of which are indicated in the patient whose myocardial infarction is complicated by heart failure and hypertension.

■ **You Should Know**

1. Beta-adrenergic blockers are contraindicated in the acute heart failure patient.

2. Nifedipine reduces ventricular contractility and, therefore, should not be given to the patient who is in heart failure.

E 047   **Answer: A and B**
A and B are correct because hypomagnesemia and hypokalemia increase myocardial sensitivity to digoxin, thus making digoxin toxicity more likely.

■ **You Should Know**

1. Digoxin toxicity is manifest as:
   a. Ectopy, both ventricular (ventricular premature beats, ventricular tachycardia), and supraventricular (atrial premature beats, atrial tachycardia).
   b. Atrioventricular block (1st, 2nd, and 3rd degree).

2. In the patient who takes digoxin, hypokalemia of any etiology predisposes to toxicity.

3. The two most common causes of hypokalemia are:
   a. Thiazide and loop diuretic therapy
   b. Diarrhea

4. Hypomagnesemia alone also predisposes to digoxin toxicity. The two most common causes of this electrolyte abnormality are:
   a. Diuretics (thiazide and loop)
   b. Chronic alcohol abuse

5. Hypomagnesemia causes prolongation of the QT interval on the electrocardiogram. Other causes of acquired long QT syndrome are hypocalcemia and medicines (e.g., phenothiazines, haloperidol, risperidone, tricyclic antidepressants, and the antihistamines terfenadine and astemizole). A long QT interval increases the risk of the patient developing polymorphic ventricular tachycardia (torsade de pointes).

6. Long QT syndrome may also be congenital. Torsade typically occurs in these children during times of sympathetic nervous system activity (e.g., during exercise or emotional stress).

E 048   **Answer: A, B, D, and E**
A and D are correct because verapamil is a smooth muscle dilator. Thus, verapamil reverses coronary artery spasm, which is the mechanism producing variant angina pectoris. Dilatation of the smooth muscle in arterioles makes verapamil effective in treatment of hypertension. B is correct because verapamil reduces frequency of migraine attacks although its mechanism of action is unknown. E is correct because verapamil slows heart rate and has a negative inotropic effect, thus making it beneficial in the patient with hypertrophic obstructive cardiomyopathy.

■ **You Should Know**

1. Verapamil is effective in therapy of variant angina pectoris that is due to coronary artery vasospasm. This medicine both relieves the acute vascular constriction and also can be used as a preventive medication.

2. Verapamil is effective in the patient who has chronic stable angina pectoris, even when spasm is not an influencing factor. Verapamil is particularly suited for the anginal patient who, concomitantly, has migraine headaches or esophageal spasm.

3. In the anginal patient who also has obstructive lung disease or claudication, verapamil is preferred in comparison to beta-adrenergic blockers. Beta blockers increase outflow air obstruction and worsen arterial claudication symptoms.

4. Verapamil is effective in terminating paroxysmal supraventricular tachycardia (PSVT), particularly when adenosine is contraindicated or ineffective. In addition, this medication may be prescribed to prevent recurrent episodes of PSVT. Important clinical point: adenosine may worsen bronchospasm.

5. Verapamil slows atrioventricular conduction and, therefore, is effective in slowing the ventricular rate in the atrial fibrillation (AF) patient. Caution: verapamil reduces ventricular contractility. Consequently, in the atrial fibrillation (AF) patient whose state is complicated by heart failure with pulmonary congestion, verapamil may worsen the heart failure. In this patient, digoxin is the preferred medication to slow the ventricular rate.

E 049   **Answer: A, B, C, D, and E**
A and D are correct because dysmorphic (abnormal-shaped) erythrocytes, red blood cell casts in the urine and/or proteinuria, suggests glomerular disease (acute glomerulonephritis and Henoch-Schönlein purpura). B and E are correct because these disorders are associated with red blood cells leaking into the urine. C is correct because the inflamed urinary bladder wall in the cystitis patient will cause hematuria.

■ **You Should Know**

1. Henoch-Schönlein purpura is the most common vasculitis in children, but it does affect adults as well. This disease commonly follows an upper respiratory infection. In addition to the renal manifestation, rash (palpable purpura), arthritis, and abdominal pain are frequent features of this illness.

2. Cystitis, renal cell carcinoma, and polycystic kidney disease are common causes of hematuria. These diseases may cause microscopic or gross hematuria.

3. The autosomal-dominant inherited polycystic disease is typically associated with hypertension, progressive renal failure, flank pain, and, often, nephrolithiasis.

E 050   **Answer: A, B, and C**
A is correct because alcohol ingestion may cause macrocytosis unrelated to folic acid metabolism. B is correct because liver disease is a common cause of macrocytosis. C is correct because hypothyroidism alone occasionally causes macrocytosis. In each of these cases the mechanism producing macrocytosis is unknown.

You Should Know

1. Megaloblastic anemia is associated with macrocytosis, but not all macrocytosis is related to a megaloblastic bone marrow.

2. Alcohol ingestion causes macrocytosis even before anemia occurs and even when body stores of folate and vitamin B_{12} are adequate.

3. Hypothyroidism is associated with an increased risk of the patient developing pernicious anemia. Pernicious anemia causes a megaloblastic bone marrow and peripheral macrocytosis.

E 051   **Answer: A, B, and C**

A is correct because there is impaired intestinal absorption of vitamin B_{12} in the patient with pernicious anemia. B is correct because vitamin B_{12} is found in food of animal origin. Therefore, patients who follow a strict vegan diet will develop vitamin B_{12} deficiency. C is correct because inflammation in the terminal ileum in some patients with Crohn's disease will cause vitamin B_{12} deficiency and megaloblastic anemia.

You Should Know

1. Intrinsic factor is essential for vitamin B_{12} to be absorbed in the distal ileum.

2. Pernicious anemia (PA) is associated with the presence of anti-intrinsic factor antibodies and anti-parietal cell antibodies. The anti-intrinsic factor antibodies prevent absorption of vitamin B_{12}. PA patients have achlorhydria.

3. Persons who follow a strict vegan diet without intake of dairy products, meat, and fish will develop vitamin B_{12} deficiency.

4. Gastrectomy will lead to deficiency of the vitamin because the stomach is the source of intrinsic factor production.

5. Vitamin B_{12} deficiency megaloblastic anemia may cause the patient to complain of paresthesias, ataxia, and sore tongue. Typical neurologic abnormalities include loss of proprioception and position sense.

6. Patients with vitamin B_{12} deficiency anemia have increased serum levels of methylmalonic acid. This serum level may be obtained when the serum vitamin B_{12} level is borderline.

7. Folic acid deficiency anemia does not cause neurologic impairment.

8. In a patient with vitamin B_{12} deficiency anemia, dietary folate will reverse the anemia but will not reverse the neurologic impairment.

9. Peripheral blood examination in the patient who has vitamin B_{12} deficiency or folic acid deficiency will show macrocytosis and hypersegmented neutrophils.

E 052   **Answer: A, B, C, and D**

A is correct because acetylcholine receptor antibodies are found in patients with myasthenia gravis, a disease that affects skeletal muscle. B is correct because Graves' disease patients typically have thyroid-stimulating hormone (TSH) receptor antibodies in the serum. C is correct because nearly all patients with Hashimoto's disease have antibodies to thyroglobulin and thyroid peroxidase. D is correct because systemic lupus erythematosus (SLE) patients typically have serum anti-nuclear antibodies.

You Should Know

1. Myasthenia gravis does not affect smooth muscle.

2. Graves' disease patients, in contrast to hyperthyroidism of other etiology, may have exophthalmos, pretibial myxedema, and periorbital and conjunctival edema.

3. Systemic lupus erythematosus (SLE) is much more common in women. Frequent symptoms include arthralgia or arthritis and chest pain due to pleuritis or pericarditis. Pericarditis may be the initial manifestation of the disease. Any female who has acute pericarditis must have systemic lupus erythematosus (SLE) ruled out.

4. Patients with systemic lupus erythematosus (SLE) often have a malar rash or a rash in sun-exposed areas. Patients should try to avoid high sun exposure and they should use sun screen agents.

5. Neurologic complications of systemic lupus erythematosus (SLE) include seizures, psychosis, and delirium.

6. Seventy-five percent of patients with untreated sarcoidosis have elevated serum levels of angiotensin-converting enzyme.

E 053   **Answer: A and B**
A and B are correct because eosinophiles are typically found in atopic tissues (tissues affected by an allergic process).

You Should Know

1. The nasal mucosa in allergic rhinitis may be pale or may be violaceous.

2. Rhinitis medicamentosa is a condition in which the nasal mucosa is inflamed from overzealous use of sympathomimetic decongestants.

3. Nasal polyposis is a potential complication of chronic allergic rhinitis.

4. The asthmatic patient who has nasal polyps should not take aspirin or traditional nonsteroidal anti-inflammatory medicines. A cyclooxygenase inhibitor medicine (COX-2 inhibitor) might be safely taken, but only after successful challenge by an allergist.

5. Intranasal corticosteroid sprays are the most effective agents in the treatment of allergic rhinitis.

E 054   **Answer: A, B, C, and E**
A, B, C, and E are correct because hydralazine, nitrates (including isosorbide dinitrate), niacin, and calcium channel blockers are all smooth muscle dilators and can cause orthostatic hypotension.

You Should Know

1. Niacin is most likely to cause hypotension when taken with other vasodilators.

2. The normal response of the body to assumption of the upright position is characterized by the following sequence: (a) decreased venous return to the right atrium; (b) decreased arterial blood pressure; (c) stimulation of the baroreceptor reflex; and (d) increase in sympathetic nervous system tone resulting in an increase in heart rate and systemic vascular resistance. Thus, with assumption of the upright position, the normal response is a small decrease in systolic pressure (5–10 mm Hg), an increase in diastolic pressure (5–10 mm Hg), and an increase in heart rate (10–20 beats/min). The change in heart rate as the blood pressure falls is an important clinical sign (see following item 5).

3. Orthostatic hypotension is characterized by a drop in both systolic and diastolic blood pressure, typically considered to be a 20 mm Hg drop in systolic pressure and a 10 mm drop in diastolic pressure in association with symptoms of decreased cerebral blood flow, namely, lightheadedness, visual blurring or darkening of the visual fields, or syncope.

4. The most common causes of orthostatic hypotension are medicines, hypovolemia, and autonomic insufficiency (sympathetic nervous system dysfunction). Medicines that commonly provoke orthostatic hypotension include hydralazine, angiotensin-converting enzyme inhibitors, nitrates, calcium channel blockers, tricyclic antidepressants, phenothiazines, and diuretics.

5. A patient who has orthostatic hypotension due to hypovolemia (e.g., blood loss or hypovolemia due to excessive diuresis or adrenal insufficiency) will have a compensatory increase in heart rate when the blood pressure drops in the standing position. In contrast, the patient who has orthostatic hypotension due to autonomic insufficiency (as commonly occurs in patients with diabetes mellitus) will have a drop in blood pressure when assuming the standing position without a compensatory increase in heart rate. Again, the heart rate response to the drop in blood pressure helps differentiate between hypovolemia and autonomic insufficiency.

E 055   **Answer: A, B, C, and D**

A, B, and D are correct because each of these conditions is characterized by thrombocytopenia. The low platelet count results in a petechial rash. C is correct because endocarditis is associated with circulating immune complexes that damage capillaries resulting in petechiae formation.

You Should Know

1. Petechiae are very tiny (pinhead) accumulations of blood that have leaked out of capillaries. They are nontender and do not blanch upon pressure.

2. Petechiae are noted on the physical examination of patients with thrombocytopenia and in certain infectious diseases in which the platelet count is normal.

3. In any disease manifest by a reduced platelet count petechiae may be found. The thrombocytopenia may be due to bone marrow disease with decreased platelet production. Alternatively, the low platelet count may be due to immunologic peripheral destruction of platelets.

4. Immunologic destruction is found in idiopathic thrombocytopenic purpura and some patient with systemic lupus erythematosus. In addition, a low platelet count is commonly noted in patients taking heparin; less commonly, sulfonamides, quinine, thiazides, cimetidine, and gold are associated with thrombocytopenia. Heparin-induced thrombocytopenia peaks at 5 to 10 days of therapy.

5. Rocky Mountain spotted fever is a rickettsial disease. Patients have the sudden onset of fever, chills, myalgia, and headache. Typically, 2 days later, a diffuse macular and petechial rash is noted, including the soles and palms. The platelet count is reduced in this disease.

6. In meningococcemia, the number and extent of petechiae are proportional to the decrease in platelet count.

7. In endocarditis, petechiae may be noted while the platelet count is in the normal range.

E 056 **Answer: A and B**

A is correct because nasal polyps are often a complication of chronic allergic rhinitis. B is correct because the majority of cystic fibrosis (CF) patients develop sinus disease and nasal polyps may be found in nearly one-third of patients.

■ **You Should Know**

1. Vasomotor rhinitis is manifest by rhinorrhea, sneezing, nasal congestion, and postnasal drip. It has no specific allergic, infectious, metabolic, or pharmacologic etiology. Symptoms are present all year long.

2. Allergic rhinitis may be seasonal or perennial.

3. Cystic fibrosis (CF) is an autosomal recessive disease with viscous secretions in ducts of the respiratory, gastrointestinal, and reproductive tracts. Respiratory involvement includes persistent cough progressing to chronic bronchitis, lung hyperinflation, bronchiectasis, and cor pulmonale. Pancreatic insufficiency and infertility are common. *Pseudomonas aeruginosa* infection is responsible for the death of the majority of CF patients.

4. In patients with nasal polyps and a history of asthma, intake of aspirin should be avoided because severe bronchospasm could result.

E 057 **Answer: A, B, and C**

A is correct because coarctation of the aorta causes hypertension. A radial-femoral pulse lag is noted on physical examination. B is correct because hypertension is common in Cushing's syndrome. C is correct because pheochromocytoma may cause episodic or chronic hypertension. Those with chronic hypertension have low plasma volume that can cause orthostatic hypotension.

■ **You Should Know**

1. Remember, a bicuspid aortic valve is very commonly found in patients who have coarctation of the aorta.

2. The pheochromocytoma patients who have paroxysmal hypertension (about half) classically have associated sweating and tachycardia.

3. A rounded face and buffalo hump are characteristic of hypercortisolism (Cushing's syndrome). Truncal obesity and purple striae are common signs. Glucose intolerance is characteristic. Hypokalemia is noted most notably when the hypercortisolism is due to ectopic adrenocorticotropic hormone (ACTH) secretion. Hypercortisolism may be due to glucocorticoid medication administration, functioning pituitary adenoma (Cushing's disease), adenoma, hyperplasia, and carcinoma of the adrenal, and ectopic adrenocorticotropic hormone (ACTH) secretion (e.g., small cell carcinoma of the lung).

4. A patient born with a bicuspid aortic valve commonly will develop severe aortic valve stenosis or regurgitation in adulthood, at approximately age 50 years.

E 058   **Answer: B, C, D, and E**
B is correct because both primary and metastatic lung cancer are associated with clubbing. C is correct because clubbing is noted in patients who have cyanotic congenital heart disease (e.g., Tetralogy of Fallot). D is correct because clubbing may occur in endocarditis, though typically late in the course of the disease. E is correct because clubbing is common in patients with long-standing cystic fibrosis.

■ **You Should Know**

1. Clubbing is not a sign of chronic obstructive pulmonary disease (COPD). If a chronic obstructive pulmonary disease (COPD) patient has clubbing, look for another cause, particularly, lung cancer.

2. Other causes of clubbing include lung mesothelioma, bronchiectasis, lung abscess, idiopathic pulmonary fibrosis, hepatic cirrhosis, and Crohn's disease of the bowel.

3. Hypertrophic osteoarthropathy (HO) is a painful condition in which there is subperiosteal formation of new bone. This causes pain in the shoulders, knees, ankles, wrists, and elbows.

4. Hypertrophic osteoarthropathy (HO) is found in patients when clubbing is due to lung cancer, mesothelioma, bronchiectasis, or cirrhosis.

E 059   **Answer: A, B, and C**
A is correct because, with increasing age, the systolic blood pressure continues to increase. This is a result of reduced compliance (or, increased stiffness) of the large arteries. B is correct because hyperthyroidism is characterized by increased pulse pressure due to the increased stroke volume and reduced systemic vascular resistance found in this disease. C is correct because chronic aortic valve regurgitation has increased pulse pressure due to the increased stroke volume increasing systolic pressure and the diastolic regurgitant flow into the left ventricle decreasing diastolic blood pressure.

■ **You Should Know**

1. With increasing age, diastolic blood pressure does not change, or may decrease. Thus, in the elderly, isolated systolic hypertension (ISH) may result.

2. Isolated systolic hypertension (ISH) increases the risk of heart failure, acute myocardial infarction, stroke, and cardiovascular mortality. It should be treated with medication.

3. The preferred initial treatment for isolated systolic hypertension (ISH) is a thiazide diuretic. A long-acting dihydropine calcium channel blocker may, alternatively, be prescribed.

4. In the elderly patient, the presentation of hyperthyroidism may be different from the younger patient. One-third of the elderly patients appear apathetic, rather than demonstrating hyperactivity and tremor. Tachycardia may be absent. However, anorexia, weight loss, and atrial fibrillation are common in the elderly hyperthyroid patient.

5. Chronic aortic valve regurgitation, with its increased left ventricle (LV) preload, leads to development of systolic heart failure.

E 060   Answer: C, D, and E
C and D are correct because pernicious anemia causes degeneration of dorsal (posterior) and lateral spinal columns. Loss of vibratory sensation and proprioception are noted on physical examination. E is correct because the Romberg test is abnormal when the patient's eyes are closed, because balance is then dependent upon proprioception sense.

■ **You Should Know**

1. The earliest neurologic abnormalities in vitamin B_{12} deficiency anemia are loss of vibratory sensation and proprioception. As the disease progresses, ataxia and weakness are noted.

2. Remember: in vitamin B_{12} deficiency, neurologic signs, even including dementia, may be present while the hematocrit and red blood cell indices are normal. The dementia is potentially reversible if the patient receives the vitamin B_{12} in timely fashion.

E 061   Answer: A, B, C, and D
A is correct because Lyme disease may affect any cranial nerve, but cranial nerve VII palsy is most common. B is correct because an unruptured cerebral aneurysm will most commonly cause cranial nerve III palsy. C is correct because 50% of sarcoidosis patients will develop cranial nerve VII palsy. D is correct because diabetes mellitus commonly causes palsy of cranial nerves III, IV, and VI, thus affecting extraocular muscle movement.

■ **You Should Know**

1. In Lyme disease involvement of cranial nerve VII may be bilateral.

2. Sarcoidosis may affect any portion of the central or peripheral nervous system.

3. Cranial nerve III palsy in the diabetic is often atypical, because pupil size often remains normal in contrast to the usual cranial nerve III palsy in which the affected eye has a dilated pupil.

4. Diabetes mellitus often causes autonomic and peripheral neuropathy. Autonomic neuropathy may cause orthostatic hypotension, gastroparesis, and retrograde ejaculation. Peripheral neuropathy is typically sensorimotor.

5. Myasthenia gravis is an autoimmune disease that affects skeletal muscle. Although ptosis is common, it is not due to cranial nerve palsy.

6. An unruptured cerebral aneurysm may cause the patient to experience facial pain, headache, or visual acuity loss even if the cranial nerve palsy is not evident.

E 062   **Answer: A, B, and C**
A is correct because the direct effect of radiation in the radioactive iodine used in treatment of the hyperthyroid patient can cause hypothyroidism to develop months or years later. B is correct because amiodarone is an iodine-containing antiarrhythmic medication that has a direct toxic effect on the thyroid gland. C is correct because lithium can cause goiter, hypothyroidism, and chronic immune thyroiditis due to its inhibition of thyroid hormone secretion.

■ **You Should Know**

1. Hypothyroidism usually develops within the first 2 years of lithium therapy. Thyroid and kidney function should be checked every 3 to 4 months in patients receiving lithium.

2. Amiodarone therapy may result in either hypothyroidism or hyperthyroidism. Thyroid function should be checked every 4 months during therapy and for 2 years afterward.

E 063   **Answer: A, B, and C**
A is correct because hypomagnesemia in the patient with alcohol abuse is due to increased renal loss of magnesium and poor nutritional intake of this nutrient. B is correct because alcohol abuse can cause a sharp fall in body folate in 4 to 5 days. C is correct because chronic alcohol abuse with its associated thiamine deficiency may cause development of Wernicke's encephalopathy.

■ **You Should Know**

1. Wernicke's encephalopathy typically has three manifestations: encephalopathy, with confusion; oculomotor abnormality, with multiple eye movement disorders including nystagmus; and ataxia due to peripheral neuropathy, cerebellar degeneration, and vestibular dysfunction.

2. Folate deficiency causes a megaloblastic anemia but does not cause the neuropathy seen in vitamin B_{12} deficiency megaloblastic anemia.

3. Chronic alcohol abuse may lead to congestive (dilated) cardiomyopathy with its associated systolic heart failure.

4. Hypomagnesemia may be due to alcohol abuse or to diuretic (thiazide or loop) therapy.

E 064 Answer: E

E is correct because in congenital long QT interval syndrome, syncope due to polymorphic ventricular tachycardia (torsade de pointes), occurs during sympathetic nervous system activation, such as occurs during exercise or emotional upset.

You Should Know

1. When asymptomatic, the long QT interval patient has a normal cardiac exam.

2. In contrast, a child with hypertrophic obstructive cardiomyopathy who faints during exercise will typically have an abnormal cardiac exam when the patient is asymptomatic. The exam may show an apical lift from left ventricular hypertrophy, a systolic ejection murmur near the apex, and a bisferiens carotid pulse.

E 065 Answer: A, B, C, D, and E

A is correct because chronic adrenal insufficiency is associated with anorexia resulting in weight loss. B is correct because nausea is common in this condition though the reason for nausea is unknown. C is correct because hyperpigmentation in Addison's disease is due to the melanocyte-stimulating effect of increased plasma adrenocorticotropic hormone (ACTH) levels. D is correct because orthostatic dizziness is due to hypovolemia from aldosterone depletion. E is correct because weakness is a common presenting symptom related to hypovolemia and electrolyte imbalance.

You Should Know

1. Primary adrenal insufficiency is most often due to autoimmune destruction of the adrenal cortex. Infectious etiologies include tuberculosis, HIV, and disseminated fungal infection.

2. Laboratory diagnosis of primary adrenal insufficiency includes low (subnormal) plasma cortisol and an elevated plasma adrenocorticotropic hormone (ACTH) level. The cosyntropin test is used in diagnosis of primary insufficiency.

3. Pigmentation in Addison's disease is most noticeable in palmar creases, friction areas, and sun-exposed areas of the skin.

4. Hyponatremia occurs in 90% and hyperkalemia in 65% of Addison's patients.

5. The hypovolemia due to the deficiency in aldosterone secretion causes hypovolemia with resultant symptomatic orthostatic hypotension.

6. Secondary adrenal insufficiency may be due to pituitary tumor or postsurgical or postradiation effects. Hyperpigmentation does not occur in secondary insufficiency. Otherwise, symptoms are the same as in primary adrenal insufficiency. In the secondary form, plasma adrenocorticotropic hormone (ACTH) is low and hyperkalemia does not occur.

E 066   **Answer: B and D**
B is correct because the increased serum alkaline phosphatase reflects the increased bone formation that occurs in Paget's disease. D is correct because the increased urinary hydroxyproline is a result of the accelerated bone resorption that is also present in this disease.

■ **You Should Know**

1. Paget's disease is often diagnosed because of asymptomatic elevation of serum alkaline phosphatase or radiologic findings that may include expanded bone that is denser than normal or has a "cotton wool" appearance.

2. Bone pain may occur in Paget's disease. The head often increases in size causing damage to cranial nerve VIII resulting in hearing loss.

3. In this disease, serum calcium and phosphorus are normal.

4. Bisphosphonates are used to treat Paget's disease.

5. Increased gamma-glutamyl transpeptidase (GGTP) levels are found in patients who have disease of the liver, biliary tract, or pancreas, but not in bone disorders. In contrast to the patient who has Paget's disease, patients with liver, biliary tract, and pancreatic disease have increased serum levels of both alkaline phosphatase and gamma-glutamyl transpeptidase (GGTP).

E 067   **Answer: A and B**
A is correct because calcium channel blockers increase capillary hydrostatic pressure. This causes fluid from the vascular space to move into the interstitium resulting in edema formation. B is correct because nonselective nonsteroidal anti-inflammatory agents (NSAIDs) cause sodium and water retention via a kidney mechanism.

■ **You Should Know**

1. Verapamil appears to cause edema less frequently than other calcium channel blockers.

2. Other medicines that may be associated with edema formation include diazoxide, minoxidil, fludrocortisone, and estrogen.

E 068   **Answer: B**
B is correct because revaccination is indicated only if the patient was under the age of 65 years at the time of initial pneumococcal vaccination and more than 5 years has elapsed or the patient is in an immunocompromised state.

■ **You Should Know**

Pneumococcal vaccine:

1. Vaccination is recommended for all adults at or after age 65 years.

2. Vaccination is recommended for younger patients who have chronic cardiopulmonary disease, diabetes mellitus, chronic alcohol abuse, chronic liver disease, or who have immunocompromised health status.

3. Immunocompromised patients would include those with HIV infection, malignancy, chronic renal disease, those on chemotherapy or corticosteroid medication, those who are asplenic (postsurgical splenectomy or autosplenectomy), and those post-organ or bone marrow transplantation. Autosplenectomy may occur in patients who have infarction of the spleen (e.g., sickle cell anemia).

4. Finally, vaccination is recommended for those who, at any age, are residents in special environments (e.g., nursing homes).

Meningococcal vaccine:

1. Meningococcal vaccine is recommended for college students who live in dormitories.

Herpes zoster vaccine:

1. Herpes zoster vaccine is recommended for adults more than 60 years of age. It is not recommended for patients with immunocompromised health status.

E 069   Answer: A

A is correct because plasma Nt-BNP levels are used in the evaluation of dyspnea, particularly in differentiation of dyspnea due to heart failure from pulmonary dyspnea. Elevated plasma levels of Nt-BNP are found in heart failure patients.

1. There are several natriuretic peptides. BNP and Nt-BNP are fragments of pro-B-type natriuretic peptide (BNP). The natriuretic hormones are released from atria and ventricles due to *stretching of the ventricles*.

2. B-type natriuretic peptide (BNP) has multiple physiologic effects, including diuresis and natriuresis (loss of sodium in the urine); it also inhibits the vasoconstrictive effect of endothelin.

3. Normal values of B-type natriuretic peptide (BNP) depend upon a number of factors. One important factor is age; B-type natriuretic peptide (BNP) levels increase threefold between the ages of approximately 40 years and 80 years.

4. The greatest value of plasma Nt-BNP appears to be its negative predictive value. In other words, a normal plasma level of Nt-BNP is excellent in excluding heart failure.

5. Elevated plasma levels of Nt-BNP are found in heart failure patients. Again, the hormone level must be correlated with the patient's age, making interpretation more difficult. Thus, a normal Nt-BNP level (<125 pg/mL) is more valuable in *excluding the diagnosis of heart failure*.

E 070   Answer: C

C is correct because a thiazide diuretic is the recommended initial agent in treating the uncomplicated hypertensive patient, that is, the patient without other medical illnesses.

■ **You Should Know**

1. Thiazide diuretics lower urinary calcium excretion. Therefore, they are preferred in patients who have recurrent urinary calcium stones. They have a beneficial effect in hypertensive patients who also have osteoporosis.

Thiazides increase serum uric acid and should not be given to patients who have gout or hyperuricemia.

2. Angiotensin-converting enzyme inhibitors (ACEI) are first-line agents in treatment of hypertensive patients who have heart failure, asymptomatic left ventricular dysfunction, history of ST segment elevation myocardial infarction, diabetes mellitus, or renal failure with accompanying proteinuria. Angiotensin-converting enzyme inhibitors (ACEI) should not be given to a pregnant woman or to a woman who is likely to become pregnant.

3. An alpha 1-adrenergic blocker may be the preferred initial antihypertensive therapy in the male hypertensive who has symptomatic benign prostatic enlargement.

4. The alpha 2a-adrenergic receptor agonist clonidine should not be stopped suddenly. It should be withdrawn over 7 to 10 days to avoid an acute hypertensive reaction.

5. A beta-adrenergic blocker or a nondihydropine calcium channel blocker may be the preferred antihypertensive therapy in the patient who has angina pectoris or atrial fibrillation.

6. A beta-adrenergic blocker may worsen manifestations of depression.

E 071   Answer: A
A is correct because isosorbide dinitrate in the man taking sildenafil may cause profound orthostatic hypotension

■ You Should Know

1. Sildenafil is a phosphodiesterase 5 inhibitor.

2. Sildenafil should not be taken by the male who is taking long-acting nitrates.

3. Sildenafil may be taken with caution by the man who also takes the alpha blocker doxazosin. It is recommended that the sildenafil be taken at least 4 hours after the last dose of the doxazosin.

4. Selective serotonin receptor inhibitors (SSRIs), spironolactone and clonidine, may cause sexual dysfunction in the male.

E 072   Answer: A, B, C, and E
A, B, C, and E are correct because bacterial and fungal infection, as well as mite infestation, can produce pustular lesions.

■ You Should Know

1. Pustules are fluid collections of white blood cells and serous fluid.

2. Rosacea is frequently found in the central face and neck. The pustules are associated with erythema and telangiectasia. Flushing episodes are common in rosacea patients. This disorder is exacerbated by alcohol and stress. Its cause is unknown. Topical application of either benzoyl peroxide or metronidazole is an appropriate initial treatment.

3. Tinea barbae is a fungal infection of the face. A potassium hydroxide (KOH) test done from material removed from the roof of the pustule or a plucked beard hair will show hyphae.

4. Impetigo is a staphylococcal or streptococcal folliculitis. The pustules may develop into honey colored crusts. A razor blade can spread the bacteria on the face. Gram stain and culture confirm the diagnosis.

5. Scabies due to mite infestation can produce pruritic pustules, papules, and vesicles. Lesions typically involve the finger webs, flexor aspects of the wrists, and male genitalia. Scrapings from the pustules, when viewed under light microscopy, may show mites, eggs or fecal material. Treatment includes bagging of recently worn clothes in a plastic bag for 1 week, then machine washing and hot drying. Systemic antibiotics may be necessary.

6. Lichen planus is a violaceous papular rash with fine white streaks on the skin and mucous membranes. Buccal involvement may be painful. The etiology is unknown. Many medicines, including nonsteroidal anti-inflammatory agents and angiotensin-converting enzyme inhibitors (ACEI) have been associated with lichen planus.

E 073   Answer: E

E is correct because pulmonary hypertension due to lung disease can cause right heart failure.

■ You Should Know

1. Cor pulmonale is heart disease secondary to lung disease. The lung disease may be vascular (e.g., multiple pulmonary emboli), or parenchymal (e.g., chronic bronchitis), pulmonary fibrosis, and pneumoconiosis. Pickwickian syndrome patients, with massive obesity and hypoventilation, may also develop cor pulmonale. **Important: alveolar hypoventilation of any etiology causes hypercarbia (i.e., elevation of systemic arterial pCO2 [$Paco_2$]).**

2. The common denominator in cor pulmonale is pulmonary hypertension that leads to right ventricular heart failure. The pulmonary hypertension is primarily due to a combination of pulmonary vascular bed obliteration and alveolar hypoxia.

3. Signs of cor pulmonale include left parasternal lift, elevated central venous pressure, congestive hepatomegaly, ascites, and peripheral edema. Chronic bronchitis, not emphysema, may progress to cor pulmonale.

E 074   Answer: A, B, and C

A, B, and C are correct because haloperidol appears to have a greater likelihood to produce extrapyramidal signs (EPS), but EPS are common as well in patients who take thiothixene or fluphenazine.

■ You Should Know

1. Extrapyramidal signs (EPS) include dystonia (abnormal movements or postures), akathisia (a desire to be in constant motion), and Parkinsonism.

2. Side effects of benzodiazepine anti-anxiety medicines are typically dose dependent. They may include ataxia, dysarthria, and poor judgment. In addition, agitation, psychosis, and confusion may occur.

3. Sertraline is a selective serotonin reuptake inhibitor (SSRI) anti-depressant that may cause somnolence, dizziness, and gastrointestinal symptoms.

4. Serotonin has central and peripheral nervous system effects. Centrally, it modulates attention and behavior. Peripherally, it influences intestinal motility, vasoconstriction, uterine contraction, and bronchoconstriction.

5. "Serotonin syndrome" is a potentially life-threatening condition most frequently related to either a high dose of the selective serotonin reuptake inhibitor (SSRI) or to a drug interaction. Drug interactions may include the selective serotonin reuptake inhibitor (SSRI) plus one of the following: amphetamine (or other adrenergic-stimulating agent), meperidine, St. John's wort, sumatriptan, and lithium.

6. Serotonin syndrome is typically manifest as agitation, delirium, vomiting, diarrhea, and sweating. Pupils are dilated; the skin is flushed; tachycardia, and fluctuating hypertension are typical signs.

E 075   **Answer: A, B, and C**
A, B, and C are correct because nonsteroidal anti-inflammatory medicines (NSAIDs) may produce gastritis and peptic ulcer. Further, they may cause interstitial nephritis and increase hypertension.

■ **You Should Know**

1. Renal effects are more common in the elderly and those taking diuretics.

2. Nonsteroidal anti-inflammatory medicines (NSAIDs) do not alter disease progression in rheumatoid arthritis, but do ease pain and inflammation.

3. Nonsteroidal anti-inflammatory medicines (NSAIDs) may precipitate heart failure due to hypertension from systemic vasoconstriction and the sodium and water retention promoted by these medicines.

E 076   **Answer: B**
B is correct because methotrexate is an anti-metabolite that interferes with cellular utilization of folic acid.

■ **You Should Know**

1. Milk reduces gastrointestinal absorption of methotrexate.

2. Methotrexate is usually the agent of choice for rheumatoid arthritis patients who do not respond to nonsteroidal anti-inflammatory medicines (NSAIDs). This medicine is also used in treatment of selected patients who have ectopic pregnancy.

3. Patients taking this medication should have liver function test determinations performed every 4 to 8 weeks. Folic acid supplement ingestion reduces the risk of hepatotoxicity.

4. Patients with liver disease should not take methotrexate. Further, patients on this medication should be strongly cautioned to avoid alcohol ingestion, because this increases the risk of medicine-induced hepatotoxicity.

E 077 Answer: A, C, and E

A, C, and E are correct because patients suffering from chronic alcohol abuse, or those taking medicines that increase P450 enzyme activity (e.g., isoniazid), are at increased risk of acetaminophen toxicity. Elderly patients also are at increased risk for acetaminophen toxicity, though the reason is not clear.

■ You Should Know

1. The specific antidote to acetaminophen is *N*-acetylcysteine. This may be given orally or intravenously to the patient.

2. Specific indications for treatment of the patient suffering from acetaminophen toxicity are outlined in a published nomogram.

E 078 Answer: C

C is correct because alcohol ingestion increases serum uric acid levels and may precipitate acute gout. Nonsteroidal anti-inflammatory medicines (NSAIDs) are the treatment of choice for acute gout.

■ You Should Know

1. 80% of primary gout patients are male.

2. Hyperuricemia in gout is due to either overproduction or underexcretion of uric acid and sometimes both.

3. Primary gout is metabolic; secondary gout is acquired and may be due to medicines (e.g., thiazide or loop diuretics, low-dose aspirin, and niacin), or to myeloproliferative diseases.

4. Early in its course, gout is intermittent and monoarticular. Later, it may become polyarticular.

5. Presence of synovial urate crystals is diagnostic. These crystals are negatively birefringent.

6. The kidney is the primary organ for uric acid excretion. To avoid uric acid–induced renal damage, the hyperuricemic patient must avoid intake of food and medicines that increase serum uric acid level, must exercise aggressive hydration, and take medicine to reduce the elevated serum uric acid level. Ingestion of meat and seafood increase serum uric acid level. Milk products reduce the risk of recurrent gouty attacks.

7. Nonsteroidal anti-inflammatory medicines (NSAIDs) are the treatment of choice for acute gout. The patient typically has a dramatic response to these agents. They should be continued for 5 to 10 days until all symptoms have resolved.

8. In a patient who has recurrent attacks of acute gout, a uricosuric agent (e.g., probenecid or sulfinpyrazone) is given if 24-hour urinary uric acid is <800

mg/day. Patients taking a uricosuric agent should take an agent to alkalinize the urine (e.g., potassium chloride). If the patient's uric acid excretion is >800 mg/day, allopurinol therapy is initiated.

9. Pseudogout, also characterized by acute arthritis, is associated with positively birefringent calcium pyrophosphate crystals in the joint. Radiography may show chondrocalcinosis in these patients.

E 079   Answer: A, B, and C

A, B, and C are correct because antibiotic prophylaxis is recommended when a procedure is associated with a significant risk of bacteremia.

■ You Should Know

1. In 2007 the American Heart Association made major revisions in its guidelines for the prevention of infective endocarditis.

2. The recommendation for antimicrobial prophylaxis is now limited to those patients with cardiac conditions with the highest risk of adverse outcome from infective endocarditis.

3. Patients at the highest risk include the following:
   a. Prosthetic heart valves
   b. A prior history of endocarditis
   c. Unrepaired cyanotic congenital heart disease
   d. Repaired congenital heart defects with prosthetic material or device during the first 6 months after the procedure
   e. Repaired congenital heart disease with residual defects at or adjacent to the site of the prosthetic device
   f. Cardiac valvulopathy (i.e., leaflet pathology with regurgitation, in a transplanted heart)

4. Antimicrobial prophylaxis is **no longer recommended** for the following:
   a. Bicuspid aortic valve
   b. Acquired mitral or aortic valve disease, including those who have undergone valve repair
   c. Hypertrophic cardiomyopathy

5. For dental, respiratory, or esophageal procedures, patients requiring endocarditis prophylaxis should take oral amoxicillin 1 hour prior to the procedure. Penicillin-allergic patients may take clindamycin, azithromycin, or cephalexin.

6. For gastrointestinal (except esophageal) or genitourinary procedures, endocarditis prophylaxis would include ampicillin plus gentamycin or vancomycin plus gentamycin.

7. Prophylaxis is not recommended for heart catheterization including balloon angioplasty, endotracheal intubation, or endodontic treatment.

E 080   Answer: B

B is correct because patients with infectious mononucleosis due to Epstein-Barr virus type 1 (EBV-1) have pharyngitis, often with tonsillar exudates, palatal petechiae, and diffuse adenopathy.

You Should Know

1. Posterior cervical adenopathy is highly suggestive of mononucleosis.

2. Saliva may remain infectious for 6 months from onset of symptoms. Patients should avoid contact sports for 4 weeks even if splenomegaly has not been present.

3. Positive heterophile agglutination (Monospot) or elevated anti-EBV titer are confirmatory. These tests usually become abnormal 3 to 4 weeks after symptom onset. EBV-specific antibody titers are indicated when Epstein-Barr infection is strongly suspected and the heterophile agglutination test is negative.

4. One third of mononucleosis patients have superimposed streptococcal tonsillitis requiring treatment with penicillin or erythromycin. Avoid amoxicillin and ampicillin because they commonly cause a rash in these patients.

5. Atypical lymphocytes appear approximately 1 week after symptom onset. Hemolytic anemia and/or thrombocytopenia may occur.

6. Uncomplicated mononucleosis cases are treated with saline gargles, acetaminophen, or other nonsteroidal anti-inflammatory agents (NSAIDs).

E 081 **Answer: A, B, and D**
A, B, and D are correct because annular lesions may occur in fungal and bacterial diseases as well as in psoriasis.

You Should Know

1. *Trichophyton rubrum* is the most common organism causing tinea corporis. Lesions tend to be few in number and are erythematous rings with central clearing. Potassium hydroxide (KOH) preparation of scales taken from lesions shows hyphae.

2. Tinea corporis may be treated with miconazole, clotrimazole, econazole, sulconazole, terbinafine, or butenafine. Betasone dipropionate with clotrimazole (Lotrisone) is not recommended.

3. Secondary syphilis, due to infection with the bacterium *Treponema pallidum*, is associated with diffuse annular lesions. The palms, soles, and mucous membranes are affected.

4. Psoriasis, typically, causes lesions on knees, elbows, and scalp. Lesions on the penis and vulva are common. The intergluteal fold may be red. Fingernails may be pitted (stippled). Pitting of nails is highly suggestive of psoriasis.

E 082 **Answer: A**
A is correct because psoriasis, typically, is associated with plaques with overlying silvery scales.

You Should Know

1. Chloroquine, lithium, and beta-adrenergic blockers may cause a psoriasis-like rash

2. 15% of psoriasis patients develop some type of arthritis, often distal, and affecting few joints (oligoarticular). Radiographic imaging generally shows

marginal erosion of bone and involvement of the phalanges reveals a "sharpened pencil" appearance. It should be noted, however, that psoriatic arthritis may take many clinical and radiographic forms.

3. In contrast, radiographic changes in rheumatoid arthritis tend to occur initially in wrists or feet. Soft tissue swelling and demineralization are early signs.

4. In the patient who has psoriasis, treatment with beta-adrenergic blockers, lithium, anti-malarials, and HMG-CoA reductase inhibitors ("statins") may worsen the rash.

5. Pitting of nails is an important diagnostic sign of psoriasis. In addition, a tan-brown discoloration of the nails may occur.

E 083   Answer: A, B, C, D, and E
A, B, C, D, and E are correct because an elevated serum amylase level is of nonspecific origin and may be due to gastrointestinal, renal, or reproductive diseases.

■ You Should Know

1. Serum amylase and lipase are elevated in patients who have renal failure due to reduced clearance of the enzymes.

2. Patients with acute pancreatitis precipitated by alcohol ingestion or by elevated plasma triglycerides commonly have normal serum amylase at the onset of symptoms.

3. The usual serum amylase determination by the laboratory does not differentiate between salivary and pancreatic origin.

4. Many medicines may elevate serum amylase levels. Examples include aspirin, codeine, estrogens, metronidazole, thiazides, and iodine-containing contrast media.

5. Several medical conditions are associated with elevated serum amylase levels. These include mesenteric infarction, ruptured ectopic pregnancy, multiple myeloma, cystic fibrosis, obstructed or perforated bowel, and pelvic inflammatory disease.

E 084   Answer: C
C is correct because decreased renal perfusion associated with the low cardiac output state of chronic systolic failure ("prerenal" disease) increases the blood urea nitrogen (BUN)/creatinine ratio.

■ You Should Know

1. The upper limit of normal for the blood urea nitrogen (BUN)/creatinine ratio is 20:1.

2. The two most common causes of renal failure are:
   a. Acute tubular necrosis secondary to ischemia (hemodynamic shock, sepsis, or cardiac arrest) or nephrotoxins (aminoglycosides, radiographic contrast media, myoglobinuria, or uric acid)
   b. Prerenal disease with decreased renal perfusion (heart failure, hypovolemia)

3. In acute tubular necrosis the ratio is normal.

4. In prerenal disease the ratio is increased.

5. Importantly, the blood urea nitrogen (BUN)/creatinine ratio is also increased in patients who:
   a. Have gastrointestinal bleeding
   b. Take medicines that interfere with protein anabolism (e.g., tetracycline or corticosteroids)
   c. Are chronically ill with loss of muscle mass

6. An increased ratio is more important clinically than a normal ratio.

7. A very low blood urea nitrogen (BUN)/creatinine ratio is found in those patients who have severe liver impairment.

E 085   **Answer: A**
A is correct because type 2 diabetes mellitus is due to a combination of tissue resistance to insulin (insensitivity to endogenous insulin) and a deficiency in response of pancreatic islet cells to glucose.

You Should Know

1. Type 1 diabetes mellitus is due to autoimmune destruction of pancreatic B (islet) cells. Circulating insulin is nearly absent, but plasma glucagon is elevated. Ninety-five percent of patients have HLA-DR3 or HLA-DR4 genes.

2. Early in the natural history of type 2 diabetes, hyperplasia of pancreatic B cells often occurs and explains the fasting hyperinsulinism and exaggerated insulin response to a glucose load. Later in the disease, the hyperinsulinism does not typically occur.

3. A waist to hip fat ratio of >0.9 is a sign of increased insulin resistance and indicative of an increased risk of diabetes mellitus.

E 086   **Answer: B**
B is correct because the metabolic syndrome is found in nondiabetic patients who, typically, have abdominal obesity and a combination of metabolic abnormalities, including insulin resistance, elevated plasma triglycerides, low serum HDL cholesterol, hypertension, and hyperuricemia.

You Should Know

1. Metabolic syndrome patients are at significantly increased risk for atherosclerotic disease.

2. In these patients it may be preferable to avoid thiazide or beta-adrenergic blocker therapy in hypertension due to their potential to worsen the dyslipidemia. Further, niacin therapy for the lipid disorder may significantly increase plasma glucose.

3. Polycystic ovary syndrome (PCOS) patients exhibit biochemical evidence of elevated testosterone, luteinizing hormone, and prolactin. These patients frequently have amenorrhea or abnormal uterine bleeding. They show insulin

resistance and hyperinsulinemia placing them at risk for type 2 diabetes. Polycystic ovary syndrome (PCOS) patients are most often hirsute with male hair distribution pattern.

E 087   **Answer: B**
B is correct because thiazide diuretics increase serum uric acid levels and, therefore, should not be given to the patient who has a history of gout or who has asymptomatic hyperuricemia.

■ **You Should Know**

1. Verapamil is particularly valuable in the patient who has hypertension in association with angina pectoris or atrial fibrillation.

2. Verapamil, diltiazem, digoxin, and beta-adrenergic blockers, may worsen tachy-brady syndrome (sick sinus) patients. All of these medicines slow atrioventricular conduction and may cause 1st degree, 2nd degree, and even 3rd degree atrioventricular block.

3. Beta-adrenergic blockers appear to worsen leg claudication via a decrease in cardiac output and inhibition of beta-2 receptor–mediated vasodilation. This appears to be most significant in the patient with moderate to severe claudication.

4. Nonelective beta-adrenergic blockers increase airway resistance by inhibiting beta-2–induced bronchodilation. Beta-1 blockers appear to cause less bronchoconstriction.

E 088   **Answer: A**
A is correct because respiratory syncytial virus is the most common infecting organism causing community acquired pneumonia (CAP) in a child under 5 years of age.

■ **You Should Know**

1. Viruses cause community acquired pneumonia (CAP) in approximately 20% of adults, but in children under age 5 years, viruses are the most common etiology of CAP.

2. CAP in the child (not infant) who is thought to have viral pneumonia (i.e., gradual onset of symptoms) preceding upper respiratory infection, diffuse auscultatory findings (rales, rhonchi) should not receive antibiotics as long as the patient is not toxic.

E 089   **Answer: A and B**
A and B are correct because chronic gastric infection and achlorhydria increase risk of gastric cancer.

■ **You Should Know**

1. Chronic *Helicobacter pylori* is a strong risk factor, increasing risk of gastric cancer 5 to 20 times.

Section 2 ▪ **Essentials Answers**   85

2. Upper endoscopy should be performed in all patients greater than 55 years who have new epigastric symptoms and anyone whose symptoms fail to respond to a short course of anti-secretory medicines.

3. Achlorhydria of any etiology (e.g., pernicious anemia) leads to a compensatory increase in serum gastrin, a potent inducer of gastric epithelial cell proliferation. This may be the mechanism by which pernicious anemia increases the risk of gastric cancer.

4. Prior Billroth II gastrojejunostomy is considered to be a risk factor as well.

E 090   **Answer: A, C, and E**
A, C, and E are correct because plague, anthrax, and tularemia are easily transmitted to humans and may have high mortality.

■ **You Should Know**

1. Anthrax produces a black eschar on exposed skin with surrounding vesicles. Inhaled spores of the gram-positive aerobic bacillus can cause pneumonia complicated by hemodynamic shock. Anthrax, naturally, is a disease of cattle, sheep, and swine. It has been used to infect humans in a purposeful (i.e., terrorist) manner.

2. Tularemia is a disease of rabbits and rodents that appears to be acquired from contact with animal tissue or aerosol inhalation. A papular lesion may be noted at the site of skin contact. Pneumonia may occur from inhalation; abdominal pain from ingestion of the organism.

3. Plague, a natural disease of rodents, is due to a gram-negative organism that may manifest as pneumonia, meningitis, or septicemia, the last causing purpura giving the historic name, "black death." If the infection occurs through the skin, then "bubos" may be noted. A bubo is an extremely painful inflammation of a lymph node with overlying skin edema.

E 091   **Answer: A is correct**
A is correct because an isotonic crystalloid solution (e.g., normal saline) will have the greatest portion of infused volume staying in the intravascular space, thus increasing blood pressure and tissue perfusion.

■ **You Should Know**

1. Vasopressors will not correct hypovolemia and may further reduce perfusion.

2. Infusion of hypotonic solutions (e.g., dextrose 5% in water or half-normal saline) will result in rapid movement of fluid from vascular to interstitial space.

3. Blood products will be started as soon as possible in the hemorrhagic patient.

4. There does not appear to be any clear advantage of colloid solutions (e.g., albumin or hetastarch) over isotonic saline.

5. A marked reduction in circulating blood volume may occur within the body, as blood or serum moves quickly from the vascular bed into a "third space." These patients then have a reduction in circulating blood volume that may lead to prerenal azotemia, shock, and acute tubular necrosis.

6. Examples of disorders that are associated with "third spacing" include major fractures (e.g., hip), severe pancreatitis, peritonitis, bowel obstruction, and crush injuries.

E 092   **Answer: B**
B is correct because blood pressure in the recumbent position may be near normal in the hypovolemic patient, but orthostatic hypotension is characteristically noted.

You Should Know

1. Hypovolemia excites the sympathetic nervous system, resulting in arteriolar and venous constriction and decreased renal blood flow. The skin is typically cool and, often, moist from sweating. Oliguria results from decreased renal blood flow and the avid sodium and water retention by the kidney.

2. When the central venous pressure (CVP) is 0, marked hypovolemia is present. Otherwise, central venous pressure (CVP) is not a good indicator of hypovolemia.

3. Elevated central venous pressure (CVP) is noted in right heart failure, constrictive pericarditis, superior vena cava syndrome, and pericardial tamponade.

4. Reduced skin turgor is noted in the hypovolemic patient when the skin of the thigh is pinched.

5. Hypovolemia is one of the causes of an increased blood urea nitrogen serum creatinine ratio. The upper limit of normal of the ratio is 20:1.

E 093   **Answer: B, C, D, and E**
B, C, D, and E are correct because panic disorder typically is associated with increased frequency of episodes in the premenstrual period and is related to other psychiatric disorders.

You Should Know

1. Panic disorder is manifest by recurrent, brief episodes of intense fear or terror occurring with physiologic manifestations (e.g., sweating and palpitations). Chest pain, smothering sensation, abdominal pain, and paresthesias are common somatic complaints.

2. 25% of patients have concurrent obsessive-compulsive disorder.

3. It is common for these patients to develop depression with increased suicide risk.

4. Sublingual lorazepam or alprazolam may be given in treatment of acute episodes.

E 094   **Answer: A and C**
A and C are correct because cirrhosis, with associated portal hypertension and hypoalbuminemia, is the most common cause of ascites. In addition, abdominal or pelvic malignancy, with peritoneal seeding, will cause ascites.

You Should Know

1. Hepatocellular carcinoma and lymphoma may cause ascites without peritoneal seeding.

2. It is suggested that the two most important tests on ascites fluid are (1) serum to ascites albumin gradient (SAAG), and (2) culture and sensitivity.

3. A SAAG gradient >1.1 g/dL indicates portal hypertension. A gradient <1.1 indicates absence of portal hypertension.

4. Culture is indicated in new-onset ascites and those with ascites who have fever, abdominal pain, azotemia, acidosis, or confusion. These are signs of *spontaneous bacterial* peritonitis (SBP).

5. Spontaneous bacterial peritonitis (SBP) must be differentiated from *secondary bacterial* peritonitis (e.g., from a complicating perforation in peptic ulcer or colonic diverticulitis).

6. Constrictive pericarditis is commonly associated with ascites. Left heart failure does not cause congestive hepatomegaly or ascites. Right heart failure is always associated with peripheral edema, but less commonly with ascites

E 095 **Answer: A and E**
A and E are correct because delayed emptying of the stomach may result in slow absorption of oral hypoglycemic medication or, in the insulin-dependent patient, a temporal imbalance between food intake and insulin administration. In both cases, the diabetic patient will appear to have lost proper control of blood sugar levels.

■ **You Should Know**

1. Gastroparesis and nocturnal diarrhea are gastrointestinal manifestations of diabetic neuropathy.

2. Gastroparesis is delayed emptying of the stomach. The patient may experience nausea, vomiting, or bloating.

3. In gastroparesis, upper endoscopy typically is normal except for the presence of residual food after an overnight fast. Gastric scintigraphy, with ingestion of a radioactive-labeled meal, is considered the optimal test for evaluating stomach emptying.

E 096 **Answer: E**
E is correct because a cyclooxygenase enzyme 2 (COX 2) inhibitor medication inhibits the vasodilation and anti-platelet aggregation effects of prostacyclin, leaving an unopposed COX-1 effect of platelet aggregation and vasoconstriction.

■ **You Should Know**

1. Cyclooxygenase (COX) enzymes produce prostaglandins, prostacyclin, and thromboxane.

2. COX-1 enzyme is responsible for platelet production of thromboxane and mucosal integrity of the stomach.

3. COX-2 enzyme is responsible for the endothelium of blood vessels producing prostacyclin. Further, COX-2 activity is increased in inflammatory states.

4. Remember, COX-1 relates to platelets and to thromboxane causing vasoconstriction and increased platelet aggregation.

5. Remember, COX-2 relates to endothelium and to prostacyclin causing vasodilation and *inhibition* of platelet aggregation.

6. As a result, COX-2 inhibitors have been found to cause increased arterial thrombosis, myocardial infarction, and stroke in patients taking these agents.

7. In contrast, nonaspirin, nonselective nonsteroidal anti-inflammatory agents (NSAIDs) inhibit *both COX-1 and COX-2*.

E 097   Answer: A, B, C, D, and E

A, B, C, D, and E are correct because the risk of adverse effects from thrombolytic therapy is increased in patients with intracranial neoplasm, uncontrolled hypertension, recent significant trauma, and active internal bleeding.

■ You Should Know

1. Thrombolytic therapy is effective in selected patients with *acute ischemic stroke* when administered within 3 hours of onset of symptoms.

2. The mechanism of action of thrombolytic medicine is to activate plasminogen resulting in degradation of fibrin in the thrombotic clot.

3. Thrombolytic therapy has an increased risk of intracerebral bleeding in the ischemic stroke patient, especially in the elderly patient. However, the benefit of therapy outweighs the relative increase in bleeding risk in this group. Those patients who have an intracranial neoplasm have increased risk of bleeding into the tumor. In this latter group, the thrombolytic agent should not be administered.

4. The thrombolytic agent may be started in the markedly hypertensive patient when the blood pressure is <170/110 mm Hg and there are no other contraindications.

5. In both acute ischemic stroke and acute myocardial infarction, patients older than age 80 years have an increased risk of intracerebral bleeding from thrombolytic agents. It is important to note, however, that the benefit of therapy outweighs the added risk.

E 098   Answer: A, B, and E

A, B, and E are correct because the pain of zoster may precede the rash for 24 to 48 hours and infection in uncomplicated cases affects a single, unilateral dermatome.

■ You Should Know

1. HIV-infected patients are much more likely to develop zoster and in these patients the infection is often generalized.

2. Zoster affecting a single dermatome does not imply an immunocompromised state or an internal malignancy.

3. Therapy early in the disease course with acyclovir, famciclovir, or valacyclovir reduces the incidence and severity of post-herpetic neuralgia.

4. Pleurodynia is a coxsackievirus infection that causes pleuritic pain in the area of the diaphragm. Patients may have headache, fever, and nausea. The length of illness is approximately 5 to 7 days.

5. Corticosteroid therapy may increase the risk of herpes zoster dissemination in an immunocompromised host.

E 099   Answer: B

B is correct because fluoroquinolones are not recommended in patients under 18 years of age because they may cause erosion of cartilage in weight-bearing joints.

■ **You Should Know**

1. Fluoroquinolones are generally more effective against gram-negative than gram-positive organisms.

2. They are generally very effective against *Escherichia coli, Moraxella, Hemophilus*, and *Campylobacter*.

3. Fluoroquinolones are used to treat epididymitis caused by enteric organisms or with negative gonococcal culture.

4. Fluoroquinolones are no longer recommended for the treatment of gonococcal infections and associated conditions (e.g., pelvic inflammatory disease), because of increasing resistance. Similarly, penicillin G and tetracycline are associated with widespread resistant strains and are no longer recommended agents.

5. For gonococcal urethritis or cervicitis, intramuscular ceftriaxone is the preferred therapy. Alternatively, parenteral ceftizoxime, cefotaxime, or cefoxitin, administered with oral probenecid, may be given. Intramuscular spectinomycin or oral azithromycin is an appropriate therapy in the penicillin-allergic patient.

6. It is cost effective to treat for coexistent *Chlamydia* infection without screening for *Chlamydia trachomatis*. Doxycycline or azithromycin may be prescribed.

7. Females should be tested for pregnancy before any tetracycline is given.

E 100   Answer: A, B, and C

A, B, and C are correct because the Mediterranean diet reduces LDL cholesterol in addition to decreasing inflammatory markers (e.g., C-reactive protein) and insulin resistance.

■ **You Should Know**

1. The Mediterranean diet is high in unsaturated oils (canola, olive), peanuts, and avocados.

E 101   Answer: E

E is correct because 10% to 20% of patients taking an angiotensin-converting enzyme inhibitor (ACEI) develop a nonproductive cough.

■ **You Should Know**

1. Angiotensin-receptor blockers are much less likely to produce a cough.

2. The angiotensin-converting enzyme inhibitor (ACEI)–induced cough generally starts within 1 week of initiation of therapy, but the onset may be delayed up to 6 months.

3. After cessation of the angiotensin-converting enzyme inhibitor (ACEI), resolution of the cough typically occurs in 1 week, but may take up to 1 month after cessation of the medication.

4. The medication-induced cough is not more common in the asthmatic patient. Further, the angiotensin-converting enzyme inhibitor (ACEI) does not exacerbate airflow obstruction in the asthmatic.

5. The heart failure patient in whom angiotensin-converting enzyme inhibitor (ACEI) therapy is initiated and then develops a cough represents an important clinical problem. The angiotensin-converting enzyme inhibitor (ACEI) may be causing the cough, but worsening heart failure itself may produce a cough due to pulmonary congestion. The clinician must use such factors as weight gain (or loss), presence (or absence) of pulmonary rales, and presence (or absence) of gallop rhythm in determining the etiology of the cough.

E 102 Answer: D

D is correct because PORT score is based upon the patient's age, comorbid conditions (e.g., heart failure, liver or renal disease), physical examination, laboratory and radiographic findings. The total point sum recommends the site of patient care.

You Should Know

1. The causative organism is not identified in nearly half of adult patients who develop community acquired pneumonia (CAP). However, *Streptococcus pneumoniae* is the most common infecting organism.

2. Other bacteria that commonly cause community acquired pneumonia (CAP) include *Hemophilus influenzae*, *Mycoplasma pneumoniae*, and *Chlamydia pneumoniae*. Common viral pathogens include influenza virus, respiratory syncytial virus, and adenovirus.

3. Sputum Gram stain should be performed in the patient whose sputum is purulent.

4. Outpatient treatment of community acquired pneumonia (CAP) may include macrolides (clarithromycin, azithromycin), doxycycline, or fluoroquinolones. These antibiotics are preferred over penicillin, because penicillin is not effective against *Mycoplasma* and *Chlamydia*.

5. Pneumonias that may be complicated by cavitation and lung abscess include those caused by *Staphylococcus aureus*, *Klebsiella pneumoniae*, *Pseudomonas aeruginosa*, and *Legionella pneumophila*.

6. Cystic fibrosis patients are prone to infection from *Staphylococcus* and *Pseudomonas*.

7. The patient who has diabetes mellitus and the patient suffering from chronic alcohol abuse are at increased risk of *Klebsiella pneumonia*.

8. In most cases, Legionnaires' disease is transmitted to humans by inhalation of the infecting organism. Showers, mist machines, and whirlpool spas have been identified as sources of infected aerosols. Chronic lung disease, smokers, and immunocompromised patients are at highest risk for developing Legionnaires' disease. Patients may be toxic with high fever, pleurisy, and

cavitary pneumonia. Azithromycin, clarithromycin, or a fluoroquinolone is appropriate therapy.

9. In a patient who has pneumonia, do not await test results before starting an antibiotic.

E 103 **Answer: A, B, C, and E**
A, B, C, and E are correct because patients with proteinuria, both diabetic and non-diabetic, have reduced progression of glomerular disease when taking angiotensin-converting enzyme inhibitors (ACEI). Angiotensin-converting enzyme inhibitors (ACEI) are used in treatment of acute and chronic systolic heart failure. Angiotensin-converting enzyme inhibitor (ACEI) therapy in the hypertensive diabetic protects against development of nephropathy. Angiotensin-converting enzyme inhibitors (ACEI) should be given early and continued indefinitely in all patients who have had an ST elevation myocardial infarction (STEMI), regardless of the left ventricular ejection fraction unless a contraindication exists.

■ **You Should Know**

1. In patients who have had ST elevation myocardial infarction (STEMI), beta-adrenergic blockers added to angiotensin-converting enzyme inhibitors (ACEI) further improve survival.

2. In patients with hypertensive heart disease, angiotensin-converting enzyme inhibitors (ACEI) promote regression of hypertrophy. Their use in other patients who have pure *diastolic* heart failure (i.e., without concomitant systolic failure), is unclear.

3. Adverse effects of angiotensin-converting enzyme inhibitors (ACEI) include hypotension, renal failure (especially in patients who have bilateral renal stenosis), cough, and hyperkalemia. Hyperkalemia is more common in the elderly, those taking potassium-sparing diuretics, and those taking non-steroidal anti-inflammatory agents (NSAIDs).

4. Angiotensin-converting enzyme inhibitors (ACEI) are contraindicated in the pregnant woman.

E 104 **Answer: A**
A is correct because squamous cell carcinoma of the lung commonly metastasizes to regional lymph nodes and causes development of pleural effusion.

■ **You Should Know**

1. The typical signs of pleural effusion are decreased tactile fremitus, dullness to percussion, and decreased breath sounds in the area overlying the effusion.

2. Pleural fluid samples should be examined for glucose, lactic dehydrogenase (LDH), protein, amylase, and differential white blood cell count.

3. An *exudative* pleural effusion is caused by pleural and lung inflammation or from movement of fluid from the peritoneal into the pleural space. An exudate has one or more of these features:
   a. Pleural fluid protein/serum protein ratio <0.5

b. Pleural fluid lactic dehydrogenase (LDH)/serum LDH ratio <0.6
c. Pleural fluid lactic dehydrogenase (LDH) >2/3 of upper limit of normal of serum lactic dehydrogenase (LDH)
d. A pleural fluid lactic dehydrogenase (LDH) >1000 IU/L is typically found in the patient with empyema

4. A *transudative* effusion occurs in the absence of pleural disease. Pleural fluid glucose is equal to plasma glucose. The white blood cell count in the pleural fluid is <1000/microL and predominantly mononuclear. Total fluid protein is usually <3.0 g/dL.

5. Causes of transudative pleural effusion include heart failure, hypoalbuminemia (cirrhosis, nephrotic syndrome), hypothyroidism, and pulmonary embolism.

6. Causes of an exudative effusion include pneumonic effusions (bacterial, fungal, and viral), malignant effusions, tuberculosis, sarcoidosis, and abdominal inflammation (e.g., abscess, pancreatitis), or abdominal malignancy.

7. A low pleural fluid glucose occurs in exudative effusions, most commonly due to pneumonia or malignancy.

8. A pleural fluid amylase level > upper limit of normal of serum amylase suggests acute pancreatitis, esophageal rupture, or lung cancer.

9. In consolidation of the lung, as in lobar pneumonia due to *Streptococcus pneumoniae*, physical signs include increased tactile fremitus and bronchial (tubular) breath sounds.

10. Paraneoplastic syndromes occur in about 15% of lung cancer patients. Small cell cancer may be associated with:
    a. Inappropriate secretion of anti-diuretic hormone (SIADH) producing hyponatremia and low serum osmolality
    b. Ectopic adrenocorticotrophic hormone (ACTH) production

11. Squamous cell carcinoma of the lung may be associated with a paraneoplastic syndrome causing hypercalcemia due to secretion of parathyroid-hormone-related-protein.

12. Remember, hypercalcemia in malignancy is most often due to osteolytic metastases, especially from breast cancer and non-small cell cancer of the lung.

E 105   **Answer: C**

C is correct because a normal serum value of D-dimer in a patient suspected of deep vein thrombosis is thought sufficient to make duplex ultrasound study unnecessary.

■ **You Should Know**

1. D-dimer, a degradation product of fibrin, is elevated in the presence of thrombus.

2. A serum level >500 ng/mL is abnormal.

3. Use of D-dimer in diagnosis of pulmonary embolism reveals good sensitivity but poor specificity. D-dimer values are abnormal in 95% of patients who have pulmonary embolism.

4. D-dimer measurement is of greater clinical value when the serum level is normal. If the D-dimer, measured by ELISA, is <500 ng/mL, embolism can be excluded with 95% accuracy.

E 106   **Answer: A**
A is correct because superficial phlebitis causes pain in the area of the inflamed vein. Induration, redness, and a palpable venous cord are typically present.

You Should Know

1. Migratory phlebitis should arouse suspicion of an underlying malignant disease.

2. Superficial phlebitis may extend into the deep venous system, resulting in deep vein thrombosis with its potential complication of pulmonary embolism.

3. Treatment of superficial phlebitis includes nonsteroidal anti-inflammatory agents (NSAIDs), local heat, and elevation. Anticoagulants are indicated when there is concomitant deep vein involvement, especially involving the deep femoral vein.

4. Chills and fever suggest an infected (suppurative) phlebitis.

5. Superficial phlebitis arising from the presence of indwelling catheters requires removal of the catheter and antibiotic administration.

6. Necrobiosis lesions are asymptomatic, typically oval yellowish plaques on the anterior legs and ankle areas. This is one dermatologic disorder associated with diabetes mellitus; another is acanthosis nigricans.

E 107   **Answer: A, B, C, and D**
A, B, C, and D are correct because high cardiac output heart failure is of diverse origin, including thiamine vitamin deficiency, hyperthyroid state, arteriovenous fistula, and Paget's disease of bone.

You Should Know

1. High-output heart failure is characterized by ventricular performance that is greater than normal, yet inadequate to meet the metabolic needs of the body. Symptoms include dyspnea and edema. Signs typically include tachycardia, bounding pulses, increased pulse pressure, rales, peripheral edema, and gallop rhythm.

2. Arteriovenous fistulas may be congenital or acquired. Acquired are usually the result of penetrating trauma (e.g., bullet wound). The direct communication between artery and vein arises as part of the healing process. The onset of high-output failure from such a wound occurs about 2 years after the injury, but may occur as early as 6 months.

3. Hyperthyroidism increases the metabolic rate that, in turn, causes a reduction in systemic vascular resistance with subsequent increase in cardiac output. Hyperthyroidism is a common cause of atrial fibrillation, especially in the elderly patient.

4. Beriberi, resulting from thiamine vitamin deficiency, may produce high-output heart failure.

5. Paget's disease of bone results in formation of arteriovenous fistulae within bone, resulting in high-output failure.

E 108 **Answer: D**
D is correct because the anion gap helps define the underlying cause of the metabolic acidosis.

■ You Should Know

1. Metabolic acidosis (MA) is characterized by low pH and low bicarbonate concentration.

2. Metabolic acidosis (MA) may be due to increased acid production in the body (lactic acidosis or diabetic ketoacidosis), to loss of bicarbonate (severe diarrhea), or less frequently, to diminished ability of the kidney to excrete acid.

3. A patient with MA has a compensatory increase in ventilation. This reduces $Paco_2$ in an attempt to normalize pH. Kussmaul breathing in the patient with diabetic ketoacidosis is an example of increased compensatory ventilation.

4. Every patient with metabolic acidosis (MA) should have an anion gap calculation in order to determine the etiology of the acidosis.

5. Anion gap = Na − (Cl + HCO3). Generally, the normal anion gap is 7 to 12 mEq/L.

6. Causes of *increased anion gap metabolic acidosis (MA)* include:
   a. Lactic acidosis due to reduced systemic perfusion and tissue hypoxia
   b. Diabetic ketoacidosis
   c. Most renal failure patients
   d. Toxic agent ingestion (e.g., ethylene glycol, methanol, or overdose of aspirin)

7. *Normal anion gap metabolic acidosis (MA)* is most commonly noted in the patient who has severe diarrhea causing marked bicarbonate loss.

8. Treatment of metabolic acidosis (MA) includes, in addition to treatment of the underlying disorder, administration of intravenous sodium bicarbonate.

E 109 **Answer: A, B, C, D, and E**
A, B, C, D, and E are correct because carpal tunnel syndrome (CTS) is common in systemic disorders. These include rheumatoid arthritis, hypothyroidism, diabetes mellitus, acromegaly, amyloidosis, and the patient on long-term hemodialysis. Systemic disorders cause bilateral carpal tunnel syndrome (CTS) with both wrists and hands involved over a short time period. Carpal tunnel syndrome (CTS) is very common during pregnancy. The symptoms disappear promptly after delivery.

You Should Know

1. Symptoms include pain, burning, and tingling in the first 2 ½ fingers and the palmar aspect of the thumb. Symptoms are *typically worse at night.*

2. Examination shows decreased sensation in the median nerve distribution. Muscle weakness and thenar atrophy appear later.

3. Tinel's sign and Phelan's sign are typically positive in carpal tunnel syndrome (CTS).

4. Treatment of the underlying disorder is the first consideration. The carpal tunnel syndrome (CTS) is treated with wrist splinting, corticosteroid injection into the tunnel, nonsteroidal anti-inflammatory agents (NSAIDs), or surgical decompression.

5. In addition to systemic disorders, carpal tunnel syndrome (CTS) occurs in those with repetitive use of the wrists.

E 110   Answer: C

C is correct because the live vaccine is recommended for healthy persons between ages 5 and 49 years.

You Should Know

1. There are two influenza vaccines in the United States: trivalent, *inactivated* vaccine and the intranasally administered trivalent *live-attenuated* vaccine.

2. Adults who receive the live-attenuated vaccine should be given 1 dose. Children between ages 5 and 8 years who have never received any influenza vaccine should receive 2 doses of live vaccine, approximately 10 weeks apart.

3. *Contraindications to live, intranasal vaccine:*
   a. Immunocompromised patients or contacts with these patients
   b. Pregnant women
   c. Patients with diabetes mellitus and chronic lung or heart disease
   d. Persons who are allergic to eggs
   e. Persons with a history of Guillain-Barré syndrome

4. Recommendations for *inactive* vaccine:
   a. Persons 50 years of age and older
   b. Residents of chronic care facilities
   c. Patients with chronic lung and heart disease
   d. Patients with chronic metabolic disorders (e.g., diabetes mellitus, renal disease, immunosuppressed states)
   e. Women who will become pregnant during the flu season
   f. Health-care workers and contacts of high-risk patients

5. The antibody response to influenza vaccine in the HIV-infected patient is related to the CD4 counts and viral load. Vaccine is recommended for all these patients.

E 111   Answer: C

C is correct because Graves' disease is the only hyperthyroid condition that is associated with exophthalmos.

You Should Know

1. The hyperthyroid state is caused by:
   a. Graves' disease, an autoimmune disease characterized by presence of anti-thyroid-stimulating hormone (TSH) receptor antibodies; only Graves' disease patients may exhibit exophthalmos and pretibial myxedema
   b. Toxic adenomas, either single or multiple
   c. Excessive exogenous thyroid hormone ingestion
   d. Thyroiditis, causing transient hyperthyroidism

2. Atrial fibrillation is associated with any cause of hyperthyroidism and is more frequent in the elderly patient.

3. A suppressed serum thyroid-stimulating hormone (TSH) level is the best test for hyperthyroidism. Only in *rare* cases of a thyroid-stimulating hormone (TSH)-secreting pituitary tumor is the thyroid-stimulating hormone (TSH) elevated.

4. Propranolol reduces tremor, sweating, and palpitations in the hyperthyroid patient.

5. Thiourea medications (propylthiouracil [PTU] and methimazole) may be given for 12 to 24 months in young adults. Propylthiouracil (PTU) is preferred in pregnant patients or those who are breast feeding. Thiourea agents are used to prepare patients for thyroid surgery and for selected patients, usually elderly or cardiac patients, who are to receive radioactive iodine (RAI) treatment.

6. Agranulocytosis may occur from the thiourea agents. It tends to occur in the first 2 months of therapy. A sore throat in the patient often heralds the onset of this blood disorder.

7. Radioactive iodine (RAI) should not be given to pregnant women. Patients given radioactive iodine (RAI) must be followed serially for the development of hypothyroidism.

8. Subacute thyroiditis (de Quervain's) is of suspected viral etiology. It is most common in young women. It is associated with painful enlargement of the thyroid, often associated with dysphagia and fever. A hyperthyroid state occurs in half of these patients and is transitory, lasting several weeks. Ultimately, most of these patients regain euthyroid status.

9. Serum thyroid-stimulating hormone (TSH) is considered to be the most sensitive test to diagnose hyperthyroidism and *primary* hypothyroidism.

E 112   Answer: A, B, C, and D

A is correct because lumbar puncture (LP) is indicated in the patient with fever, headache, and altered mental status. The lumbar puncture (LP) may help to differentiate bacterial from viral meningitis. B is correct because lumbar puncture (LP) is important in the patient with suspected subarachnoid hemorrhage when CT imaging is negative. C is correct because the cerebrospinal fluid (CSF) in multiple sclerosis (MS) often shows lymphocytosis and slightly increased protein level. Elevated level of cerebrospinal fluid (CSF) IgG is noted in many MS patients. D is correct because the Guillain-Barré patient has increased protein with normal cell count in the cerebrospinal fluid (CSF).

■ **You Should Know**

1. The finding of xanthochromic cerebrospinal fluid (CSF) is an important indicator of earlier bleeding (as opposed to a traumatic tap causing red cells in the cerebrospinal fluid [CSF]).

2. Complications of a lumbar puncture (LP) include headache, infection, bleeding, and cerebral herniation. Headache typically occurs 24 to 48 hours after the procedure and may be frontal or occipital. Headache is increased in the upright and lessened in the recumbent position. These patients may also have nausea, vomiting, dizziness, and visual symptoms.

3. Treatment of the lumbar puncture (LP)-related headache includes epidural blood patch, bedrest, and analgesics.

4. Herniation due to increased intracranial pressure is the most serious complication. Those at greatest risk are patients with focal neurologic signs or papilledema.

5. Preferably, CT imaging is performed before a lumbar puncture (LP). However, neurologists may opt to perform lumbar puncture (LP) without prior CT imaging in selected patients who are suspected of having bacterial meningitis.

6. Contraindications to lumbar puncture (LP) include:
   a. Increased intracranial pressure
   b. Bleeding diathesis (e.g., thrombocytopenia)
   c. Spinal epidural abscess

7. Guillain-Barré syndrome is an ascending inflammatory disease of the nervous system, often following *Campylobacter* infection. The patient often has symmetrical neurologic symptoms, including paresthesias of the feet and weakness of the legs. The weakness may proceed in cephalad direction. Loss of deep tendon reflexes is typical.

E 113 **Answer: A, B, C, D, and E**

A, B, C, D, and E are correct because norovirus, rotavirus, *Giardia*, enterotoxic *Escherichia coli* and *Staphylococcus aureus* enterotoxin cause infectious, noninflammatory diarrhea.

■ **You Should Know**

1. Acute infectious diarrhea is divided into two categories:
   a. Noninflammatory, with symptoms related to the small bowel (i.e., cramps and nonbloody diarrhea)
      (1) Organisms include norovirus, rotavirus, *Giardia*, *Cryptosporidium*, *Staphylococcus aureus* enterotoxin, and enterotoxigenic *Escherichia coli*
   b. Inflammatory, with symptoms related to the colon (i.e., bloody diarrhea)
      (1) Invasive organisms include *Entamoeba histolytica*, *Shigella*, *Campylobacter*, *Salmonella*, *Yersinia*

2. Outbreaks of diarrhea at a common location (e.g., cruise ship or school), suggest viral infection or toxic food source. Norovirus affects all age groups and is a major cause of epidemic diarrhea. This is the primary etiology of nonbacterial gastroenteritis in the United States. Restaurants, long-term care

facilities, cruise ships, and day-care centers are frequent venues of infection. Fecal-oral route is the primary route of infection.

3. Unpurified water exposure suggests *Giardia* or *Cryptosporidium* infection. *Giardia* infection is commonly due to drinking mountain water when camping or swimming. *Giardia* is primarily water borne, but may be food borne when contaminated, uncooked food is eaten. Patients with giardiasis may be asymptomatic or have diarrhea. Stool microscopy looking for cysts and trophozoites is performed. Fecal antigen tests may be more sensitive. Metronidazole is the preferred therapy.

4. *Cryptosporidium* infection, causing noninflammatory diarrhea, is, considered the leading cause of recreational water-associated outbreaks of diarrhea.

6. Recent travel suggests **travelers' diarrhea.** This is most commonly due to bacterial infection, frequently with enterotoxigenic *Escherichia coli, Shigella* species or *Campylobacter jejuni*, though other organisms may be causative. This is usually benign and self-limited. Typically, stools are loose and the patient has cramps and, occasionally, vomiting. Fever is rare. For those patients traveling to high-risk areas, prophylaxis is recommended for those who have irritable bowel syndrome, AIDS, diabetes mellitus, or who are taking immunosuppressive medication. Norfloxacin, ciprofloxacin, ofloxacin, or trimethoprim-sulfamethoxazole may be taken. For healthy patients, prophylaxis against traveler's diarrhea is not recommended. However, patients may be given a supply of antimicrobial medication to be taken if needed.

7. Watery, nonbloody diarrhea with cramps, nausea, or vomiting suggests a small bowel source caused by a toxin (*Staphylococcus aureus* or enterotoxigenic *Escherichia coli*), viral infection, or *Giardia*. Tissue invasion does not occur; therefore, leukocytes are not found in the feces.

8. AIDS patients commonly have enterocolitis related to bacteria (e.g., *Campylobacter, Shigella, Salmonella*), viruses and protozoa (e.g., *Cryptosporidium, Entamoeba histolytica, Giardia*). HIV patients are likely to demonstrate more serious symptoms, including bacteremia.

9. *Campylobacter* enterocolitis, in contrast to *Giardia*, is frequently associated with high fever and chills. *Campylobacter* infection is noted to be an antecedent infection in patients who develop Guillain-Barré syndrome.

10. **Note:** *Campylobacter* may be associated with benign travelers' diarrhea or with a much more toxic state, enteritis. In enteritis, fever is present.

E 114   Answer: A and C
A is correct because bloody diarrhea is the key manifestation of ulcerative colitis. C is correct because rectal inflammation causes the patient to experience fecal urgency.

■ **You Should Know**

1. Ulcerative colitis (UC), a disease of unknown cause, is characterized by intermittent flare-ups and remissions.

2. Extent of colonic involvement in ulcerative colitis (UC) is variable, with some patients having only proctosigmoiditis, others with limited left-sided colitis, and others with extensive disease.

3. Diagnosis is established by sigmoidoscopy.

4. Colonoscopy should not be performed in patients with severe disease because of risk of perforation or inducing megacolon.

5. Patients with proctitis may be treated with mesalamine suppositories or hydrocortisone foam.

6. Patients having more extensive involvement are treated with sulfasalazine or mesalamine tablets or balsalazide. Corticosteroids are reserved for those suffering from severe disease.

7. Relapses are common. Therefore, long-term therapy with sulfasalazine or olsalazine or mesalamine is recommended. Selected patients may require an anti-TNF (tissue necrosis factor) agent or an immunosuppressive medication.

8. Extraintestinal complications include uveitis, skin disorders (e.g., erythema nodosum or pyoderma gangrenosum), large joint arthritis, and cholangitis.

9. Ulcerative colitis patients have an increased risk of colon cancer.

10. Nonaspirin, nonselective NSAIDs can produce a clinical illness similar to ulcerative colitis, with gross bleeding and diarrhea.

E 115 Answer: A, B, and C

A, B, and C are correct because, in addition to the classic symptom of heartburn, gastroesophageal reflux can cause hoarseness, water brash, and wheezing.

You Should Know

1. The classic symptom of gastroesophageal reflux is heartburn, most frequently occurring about an hour after meals and also during recumbency. Other symptoms include water brash (hypersalivation, "foaming"), sour taste in the mouth, dysphagia, hoarseness, wheezing, sore throat, and chest pain.

2. Upper endoscopy is normal in half of patients who have reflux. In selected patients, ambulatory esophageal pH monitoring is performed. This is considered the best procedure to document reflux.

3. Some patients with chronic reflux will develop Barrett's esophagus in which the squamous epithelium of the esophagus is replaced by columnar epithelium. Barrett's esophagus may lead to stricture or, more seriously, adenocarcinoma.

4. Many patients can be treated empirically. If the patient does not properly respond, further investigation is warranted.

5. Principles of general medical treatment of reflux:
   a. Do not lie down for at least 2 hours after a meal
   b. Elevate head of bed
   c. Avoid acidic foods (e.g., colas, red wine, orange juice)
   d. Avoid fatty foods, peppermint, chocolate
   e. Avoid alcohol intake and smoking

6. Medicinal treatment:
   a. For occasional symptoms: H2-receptor antagonists (e.g., cimetidine, ranitidine, or nizatidine)

b. For reflux causing symptoms several times per week: the above H2-receptor antagonists or proton pump inhibitors, omeprazole, rabeprazole, esomeprazole.

7. Reflux is a trigger of asthma. Some of these patients may not have reflux symptoms. In addition, aspiration may cause acute wheezing in the nonallergic patient. If refluxed gastric contents are in contact with the pharynx, laryngitis and hoarseness may be noted.

8. Other patients with reflux may have persistent cough. Again, some of these patients with reflux may have cough without associated heartburn or sour taste in the mouth.

E 116   Answer: C

C is correct because malignancy, especially lung, pancreas, prostate, kidney, and colon, is a risk factor for deep vein thrombosis.

You Should Know

1. In 80% of cases, deep vein thrombosis (DVT) is thought to arise in the veins of the calf. Half of these patients may have no symptoms or signs. Others may show evidence of tenderness, overlying erythema, and a palpable venous cord.

2. In addition to trauma and surgery (especially orthopedic, major vascular, and cancer surgery), malignancy is a risk factor for deep vein thrombosis (DVT).

3. In addition, a hypercoagulable state (e.g., Factor V Leiden mutation, deficiency in protein C or S, or antithrombin III) may lead to deep vein thrombosis (DVT).

4. Duplex ultrasonography is the preferred initial diagnostic test.

5. Treatment of deep vein thrombosis (DVT):
   a. Heparin, followed by warfarin, the latter for 3 to 6 months for the first episode of uncomplicated deep vein thrombosis (DVT)
   b. Indefinite warfarin therapy is recommended for those with recurrent deep vein thrombosis (DVT) or a hypercoagulable state
   c. In a patient who has had a pulmonary embolism, duration of warfarin anticoagulation depends upon whether this is a first or recurrent embolus and whether an identifiable risk factor, reversible or irreversible, has been identified

6. Oral contraceptive agents should not be given to women who smoke because of increased risk of venous thrombosis.

7. Venous thrombosis in a patient who has experienced recurrent spontaneous abortions suggests antiphospholipid syndrome.

E 117   Answer: D

D is correct because *horizontal* ST segment depression is probably the most specific sign of subendocardial myocardial ischemia.

■ You Should Know

1. It is the subendocardial layer of the myocardium that is most susceptible to insufficient perfusion (ischemia). Subendocardial ischemia (SEI) is characterized on the electrocardiogram by horizontal ST segment depression or by downward sloping (toward the end) of the ST segment. The T waves may remain positive or may become negative.

2. J point depression followed by an upsloping ST segment may represent subendocardial ischemia (SEI), but is nonspecific.

3. Changes in T waves are an unreliable indicator of myocardial ischemia. Subendocardial ischemia (SEI) may be associated with symmetrical T wave inversion, usually in association with ST segment depression. However, T wave inversion is less sensitive and less specific than ST segment depression.

4. Nonspecific ST-T abnormalities (NSSTTA) relate to slight ST segment depression or T wave inversion or T wave flattening that occurs without evident cause. Nonspecific ST-T abnormalities (NSSTTA) may occur in healthy persons, especially shortly after eating, in patients who have either acidosis or alkalosis, in patients who are febrile or anemic, in those who are in a state of heightened adrenergic tone, or in patients who have myocarditis or pulmonary embolism.

E 118   Answer: B, C, D, and E

B and D are correct but the reason is unclear. C is correct because genetic factors are thought to play a role in susceptibility to preeclampsia. E is correct because antiphospholipid antibodies produce a hypercoagulable state that causes development of preeclampsia.

■ You Should Know

1. There are four defined hypertensive disorders in pregnancy:
   a. Preeclampsia
   b. Preexisting hypertension (chronic hypertension)
   c. Preeclampsia superimposed upon preexisting hypertension
   d. Gestational hypertension

2. Preeclampsia is defined as new-onset hypertension and proteinuria after 20 weeks of gestation in a woman who was previously normotensive.

3. Other risk factors for preeclampsia include pregestational diabetes mellitus, multiple gestation, obesity, preexisting hypertension, collagen vascular disease, and renal disease.

4. Severe preeclampsia is characterized by the presence of central nervous system symptoms (e.g., blurred vision or severe headache), hepatocellular injury, and thrombocytopenia, superimposed upon the hypertension and proteinuria of mild preeclampsia.

5. Eclampsia refers to the onset of grand mal seizures in the woman with preeclampsia.

6. Endothelial dysfunction in the pregnant woman is considered to be the pathophysiologic abnormality accounting for the clinical features of the disorder.

7. The definitive treatment of preeclampsia is delivery of the infant because this condition is reversible.

8. Gestational hypertension is new-onset hypertension developing after the 20th week of gestation and not associated with proteinuria. Blood pressure typically returns to normal by the 12th week postpartum.

9. Anti-phospholipid antibody syndrome (APS) is characterized by a hypercoagulable state predisposing to arterial and venous thrombosis. Recurrent fetal loss after the 1st trimester is common. Anti-phospholipid antibody syndrome (APS) may be primary or related to systemic lupus erythematosus.

E 119   Answer: E
E is correct because transvaginal ultrasonography is valuable in detecting the presence of a gestational sac. Ultrasonography is preferred to MRI scans, culdocentesis, laparoscopy, and curettage.

■ You Should Know

1. The diagnosis of ectopic pregnancy (EP) is based upon quantitative assay for human chorionic gonadotropin (hCG) and findings on transvaginal ultrasonography.

2. Clinical manifestations of ectopic pregnancy (EP), occurring 6 to 8 weeks after the last menstrual period, are amenorrhea, vaginal bleeding, and abdominal pain.

3. However, these three manifestations are also common in threatened abortion. Transvaginal ultrasonography imaging is the most important diagnostic modality in differentiating ectopic pregnancy (EP) from threatened abortion.

4. Signs of ectopic pregnancy (EP) are highly variable. Therefore, the diagnosis is based upon human chorionic gonadotropin (hCG) concentration and imaging study.

5. Risk factors for ectopic pregnancy (EP) include:
    a. Previous ectopic pregnancy (EP)
    b. Previous tubal pregnancy
    c. History of bilateral coagulation sterilization
    d. Current intrauterine device usage
    e. In utero estrogen exposure
    f. Pelvic inflammatory disease with salpingitis

6. Treatment of ectopic pregnancy (EP) includes surgical removal or, in selected cases, administration of methotrexate.

E 120   Answer E
E is correct because HBsAg appears in serum 1 to 10 weeks after exposure to the virus and an IgM antibody is present during acute infection.

■ You Should Know

1. Serologic markers for hepatitis B virus infection (HBV) include:
    a. Hepatitis B surface antigen (HBsAg) that is detected by radioimmunoassay (RIA) or enzyme immunoassay (EIA). This marker is no

longer detectable after 4 to 6 months in those who recover. Persistence of HBsAg after 6 months indicates chronic infection.
   b. Hepatitis B surface antibody (anti-HBs). This persists for life, thus conferring long-term immunity. In hepatitis B infection, anti-HBs appears after disappearance of HBsAg.
   c. Hepatitis B core antibody (anti-HBc). This is, primarily, an IgM antibody present during acute infection. Anti-HBc may persist in the serum for 2 years after acute infection.

2. Hepatitis B core antigen (HBcAg) is not detectable in serum. It is an intracellular antigen in infected liver cells.

3. A template of selected hepatitis B panels:

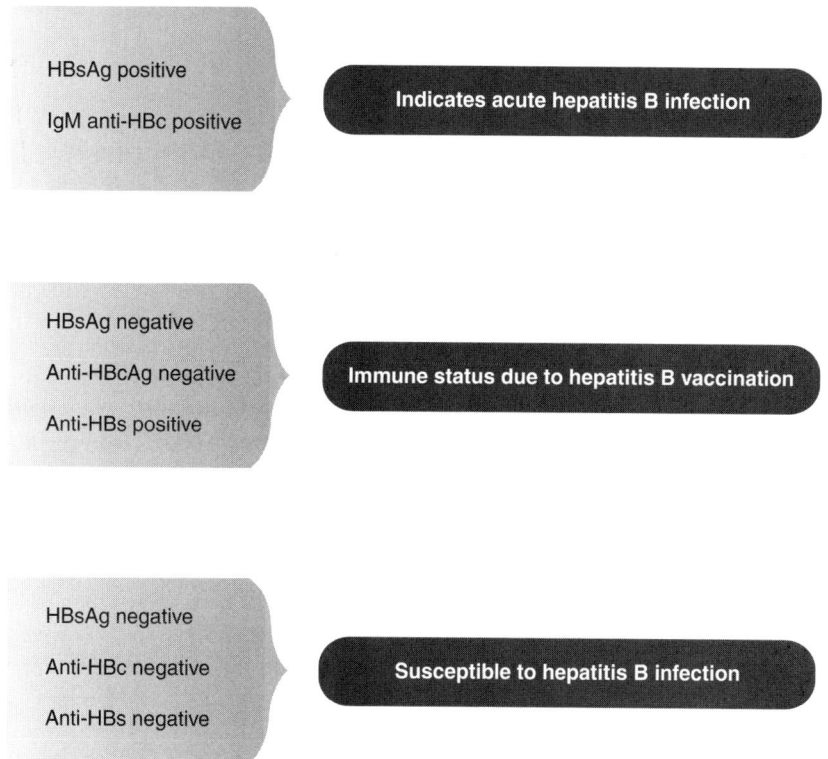

E 121   **Answer: E**
E is correct because a low birth weight baby is considered a very controversial indication for cesarean delivery.

You Should Know

1. Those considered to be the most important indications for cesarean delivery include:
   a. Failure to progress in labor
   b. Fetal distress
   c. Previous cesarean delivery or hysterotomy
   d. Fetal malpresentation (breech or transverse lie)

2. Neural tube defects and hydrocephalus are other very controversial indications.
3. Relaxation of the lower esophageal sphincter and the increased intraabdominal pressure of pregnancy predispose to gastric aspiration. Therefore, solid food should not be ingested for at least 6 hours and clear liquids for at least 2 hours before elective cesarean delivery.
4. A single dose of an antibiotic (e.g., ampicillin, cefazolin, cefotetan, or cefitoxin) is recommended immediately after cord clamping.
5. Before an elective cesarean delivery the following are indicated:
   a. Assessment of fetal lung maturity
   b. Maternal blood type and antibody screen
6. Fetal heart rate patterns are considered reassuring or nonreassuring.

Reassuring patterns include:
   a. Baseline fetal heart rate (110 to 160 beats per min)
   b. Absence of fetal heart rate decelerations
   c. Normal fetal heart rate variability (6 to 25 beats per min)

Nonreassuring patterns include:
   a. Abnormal variability in heart rate
   b. Late decelerations
   c. Sinusoidal heart rate (i.e., a pattern of regular variability considered due to fetal hypoxemia)
   d. Variable decelerations

Nonreassuring heart rate patterns must be promptly addressed and a determination whether operative intervention in the pregnancy is indicated.

7. A contraction test is usually performed using an oxytocin solution. A positive test is characterized by presence of late decelerations in fetal heart rate following 50% or more of contractions.

E 122 Answer: B

B is correct because endoscopic retrograde cholangiography permits stone extraction or stent placement in the common bile duct in this patient who has cholangitis. Patients with cholangitis have an obstruction in the common bile duct, most commonly by stones, less frequently by benign stricture.

You Should Know

1. The clinical picture of right upper quadrant or epigastric pain, fever with chills, and jaundice suggests cholangitis. Ciprofloxacin is an effective antimicrobial. Alternatively, mezlocillin plus either metronidazole or gentamycin, or both, may be administered.
2. In evaluation of the patient with jaundice, first determine whether the hyperbilirubinemia is associated with normal or abnormal liver enzymes.
3. Jaundice with normal liver enzymes:
   a. Elevated unconjugated ("indirect"): think of hemolysis, resorption of a hematoma, Gilbert's syndrome
   b. Elevated conjugated ("direct"): think of Dubin-Johnson syndrome

4. Jaundice with abnormal liver enzymes is due to elevated serum conjugated bilirubin concentration. The abnormal liver enzymes may indicate hepatocellular, cholestatic, infiltrative disease or mechanical biliary obstruction.

5. In hepatocellular disease elevation of serum alanine aminotransferase (ALT) and aspartate aminotransferase (AST) is disproportionate to increases in serum alkaline phosphatase and gamma-glutamyl peptidase (GGT). Hepatocellular disease may be due to infection, alcohol, toxins (e.g., medicines, illicit drugs, herbal preparations), or autoimmune disease. In alcoholic hepatitis the serum aspartate aminotransferase (AST)/alanine aminotransferase (ALT) ratio is often greater than 2:1.

6. Cholestatic jaundice is characterized by disproportionate increase in serum alkaline phosphatase and gamma-glutamyl peptidase (GGT) compared to aminotransferases. Cholestasis may be intrahepatic as seen in primary biliary cirrhosis or due to medicines (e.g., acetaminophen, penicillins, chlorpromazine, rifampin, trimethoprim-sulfamethoxazole), anabolic and estrogenic steroids, or in primary sclerosing cholangitis that is associated with inflammatory bowel disease. Intrahepatic cholestasis is also present in infiltrative disease of the liver (e.g., due to the granulomatous diseases tuberculosis and sarcoidosis).

7. Mechanical biliary obstruction may be due to benign disease (e.g., stone), parasitic disease (ascariasis) or malignancy (carcinoma of the pancreas or gallbladder, ampullary carcinoma, or cholangiocarcinoma).

8. Anti-mitochondrial antibody testing is highly sensitive and specific for primary biliary cirrhosis.

9. Anti–smooth muscle antibodies, anti-nuclear antibodies, and elevated serum globulins are commonly found in patients with autoimmune hepatitis. This disease usually occurs in young to middle-aged women.

E 123 Answer: E

E is correct because prostaglandin F 2-alpha (PGF2) and prostaglandin E 2 (PGE 2) stimulation of uterine contraction causes uterine ischemia. This is considered to be the cause of the abdominal cramping that typically occurs just before or with onset of menstrual bleeding.

■ You Should Know

1. Dysmenorrhea is characterized as primary dysmenorrhea (PD), (i.e., menstrual pain in absence of pelvic disease) or secondary.

2. Secondary dysmenorrhea may be due to causes including endometriosis, adenomyosis, or leiomyomata of the uterus, and pelvic inflammatory disease.

3. Primary dysmenorrhea (PD) only occurs during ovulatory cycles.

4. Treatment of primary dysmenorrhea (PD) includes application of heat to the lower abdomen, physical exercise, NSAIDs, often starting with ibuprofen and then, if necessary, mefenamic acid, or meclofenamate. To those desiring contraception, combination estrogen-progestin is indicated.

E 124 Answer: B, C, and E

B, C, and E are correct because premenstrual dysmorphic disorder is a more severe form of premenstrual syndrome (PMS) in which hopelessness, lability of mood, and anger are prominent affective symptoms.

■ You Should Know

1. Premenstrual syndrome (PMS) is manifest by repetitive physical and behavioral symptoms that occur in the second half (luteal phase) of the menstrual cycle.

2. Premenstrual syndrome (PMS) symptoms are multitudinous and include fatigue, bloating, edema, irritability and inability to concentrate.

3. In therapy of premenstrual dysmorphic disorder, gonadotropin releasing hormone (GnRH) agonists are less effective for depressive symptoms than for irritability. Other treatments include danazol, diuretics, and anti-depressants.

E 125 Answer: B

B is correct because histologic analysis for *Helicobacter pylori* is preferred in patients who have active gastrointestinal bleeding.

■ You Should Know

1. Serologic tests are less frequently used in the diagnosis of *Helicobacter pylori* infection because they are less accurate than a fecal antigen immunoassay and a C13 urea breath test.

2. Proton pump inhibitors significantly reduce the sensitivity of urea breath tests and fecal antigen assay. These medicines may cause false-negative results. Therefore, they should be discontinued 10 to 14 days before testing. However, these medicines do not affect serologic tests.

3. Gastric biopsy specimens can be tested for active infection by urease production. Histologic analysis of gastric specimens is valuable in those who are taking proton pump inhibitors.

4. Confirmation of *Helicobacter pylori* eradication can be done using either the urea breath test or stool antigen testing.

E 126 Answer: E

E is correct because ceftriaxone is a third-generation cephalosporin that is not appropriate therapy for *Helicobacter pylori*. Ceftriaxone is the treatment of choice for penicillin-resistant gonococcal infections and meningitis due to ampicillin-resistant *Haemophilus influenza*.

■ You Should Know

1. *Helicobacter pylori* is a gram-negative rod that resides in the submucosal layer of the stomach causing gastritis. This infection also is present in the majority of non–NSAID-induced duodenal ulcers.

2. Treatment options for active *Helicobacter pylori*-associated ulcer include:
   a. Proton pump inhibitor, clarithromycin, and amoxicillin
   b. Proton pump inhibitor, bismuth subsalicylate, tetracycline, and metronidazole
   c. Ranitidine, bismuth citrate, clarithromycin, and amoxicillin

E 127   **Answer: A**

A is correct because infused 0.9% saline (normal saline) remains in the extravascular space thus increasing circulating plasma volume and blood pressure. Sodium does not enter cells. It is the osmotic effect of the sodium that keeps water in the extravascular space.

■ **You Should Know**

1. Normal saline (or Ringer's lactate in the patient not in acidosis) should be the initial treatment of hypovolemic shock not due to anemia or hemorrhage.

2. In the patient being treated for diabetic acidosis: when dehydration has been corrected with normal saline infusion, evaluate serum sodium concentration. If sodium is high, change the infusion to 0.45%; if sodium is low, continue normal saline.

3. Insulin therapy in ketoacidosis: regular insulin administration by continuous intravenous infusion is the treatment of choice. Insulin therapy may be delayed if the initial serum potassium concentration is <3.3 mEq/L until replenishment elevates the potassium level to >3.3 mEq/L.

4. Patients with diabetic ketoacidosis need potassium replacement because of high urinary potassium losses during polyuria. Serial serum potassium values should be determined every 2 hours. If the arterial pH is <6.9, sodium bicarbonate in water may be given intravenously.

5. Hyperglycemic hyperosmolar state (HHS) is characterized by hyperglycemia (>600 mg/dL), serum osmolality >310 mOsm/kg but with a normal anion gap and normal systemic arterial pH. Serum bicarbonate is generally in the 15 to 20 mEq/L range. Prerenal azotemia due to severe hypovolemia may occur in these patients causing development of severe azotemia (blood urea nitrogen (BUN) levels nearly 100 mg/dL).

6. Hyperglycemic hyperosmolar state (HHS) is most frequently noted in middle-aged and elderly patients with mild diabetes mellitus. Hyperglycemic hyperosmolar state (HHS) is frequently precipitated by infection (pulmonary or urinary), acute myocardial infarction, stroke, or recent surgery. Hyperglycemic hyperosmolar state (HHS) patients typically present with polyuria, polydipsia, and weakness. Confusion and coma may occur.

7. Hyperglycemic hyperosmolar state (HHS) therapy includes intravenous insulin, intravenous fluids (0.9% saline initially), and potassium replacement.

E 128   **Answer: A**

A is correct because metformin tends to cause less weight gain than other hypoglycemic agents and, thus, is preferred therapy in the obese diabetic.

You Should Know

1. Sulfonylureas are a reasonable first-line choice of therapy in type 2 diabetes mellitus patients who are minimally overweight.
2. Avoid metformin therapy if serum creatinine concentration is greater than 1.4 mEq/L in women or greater than 1.5 mEq/L in men, in patients with decompensated heart failure, those with liver failure, or with heavy alcohol intake. The risk of lactic acidosis is increased in these patients.
3. A patient receiving metformin therapy should not take the medication on the day in which an intravenous radiocontrast agent is received and for 2 days thereafter. This is to avoid lactic acidosis if renal insufficiency occurs.
4. Type 2 diabetes mellitus patients who have hypertension must be aggressively treated. Blood pressure target is <130/80 mm Hg.
5. The "dawn phenomenon" is associated with rapidly rising plasma glucose levels between 3 AM and 8 AM. It occurs in type 1 diabetes patients when the plasma insulin level is low due to complete absorption of the prior evening's insulin dose at the time (early AM) when there is an increased need for insulin (due to morning release of growth hormone, which antagonizes the action of insulin).

E 129 Answer: E

E is correct because amantadine is not recommended therapy because of the high number of resistant influenza viral strains.

You Should Know

1. Acute bronchitis in healthy persons is usually due to viral infection. The bronchitis due to influenza typically is associated with constitutional symptoms (e.g., fever, myalgia, prostration).
2. Viral bronchitis due to such organisms as coronavirus, rhinovirus, and respiratory syncytial virus typically do not have associated constitutional symptoms. Much less frequently, acute bronchitis is due to *Chlamydia*, *Mycoplasma*, or *Bordetella*.
3. Treatment of acute viral bronchitis in the adult includes an analgesic (NSAID, aspirin, acetaminophen), decongestants, bronchodilators, increased fluid intake and, occasionally, a cough suppressant. Antibiotics are not recommended as routine treatment of acute bronchitis.
4. Influenza A and B produce the same clinical symptoms. Therapy with oseltamivir or zanamivir are of value when started within 48 hours of symptom onset.

E 130 Answer: B and E

B is correct because loop diuretics and thiazide diuretics may cause hypokalemia due to increased urinary potassium excretion. E is correct because alkalosis of any etiology causes hydrogen ions to come out of cells into the blood. As a result, potassium moves from serum into cells resulting in hypokalemia.

You Should Know

1. Common symptoms associated with hypokalemia include weakness, muscle cramps, and fatigue.

2. The electrocardiographic manifestations of hypokalemia are flattening of the T wave, prominence of the U wave, and ST segment depression.

3. Beta 2-adrenergic agonists promote cellular uptake of potassium. Therefore, nebulized albuterol is a treatment for hyperkalemia. Other treatment options for hyperkalemia include intravenous calcium gluconate, intravenous insulin in glucose solution, and sodium bicarbonate.

4. Angiotensin-converting enzyme inhibitor (ACEI) therapy tends to increase serum potassium due to reduced aldosterone secretion. Patients at increased risk of hyperkalemia from angiotensin-converting enzyme inhibitors (ACEI) therapy include those with diabetes mellitus, renal insufficiency, hypovolemia, or those with concurrent intake of potassium-sparing diuretics or NSAIDs.

5. Intravenous lidocaine is used to treat ventricular ectopy in the setting of acute myocardial infarction. Neurologic toxicity is the most common adverse effect of the medicine; the symptoms always resolve with discontinuation of the drug. Side effects include tremor, insomnia or drowsiness, slurred speech, change in sensorium, and hallucinations. Generalized seizures may occur. Lidocaine side effects are more common in the elderly and those with heart failure or liver impairment.

E 131 Answer: A

A is correct because patients with myasthenia gravis typically have one of several subtypes of antibodies to acetylcholine receptors.

■ You Should Know

1. Myasthenia gravis is a disease affecting skeletal muscles. It does not affect smooth muscle.

2. Graves' disease patients have autoantibodies to the thyroid-stimulating hormone (TSH) receptor. Antibodies are not characteristic of other diseases causing hyperthyroidism.

3. Nearly all patients with Hashimoto's thyroiditis have antibodies to thyroglobulin and thyroid peroxidase.

4. In 70% of pernicious anemia patients anti-intrinsic factor antibodies are present. Less frequently, these patients have anti-parietal cell antibodies.

5. Anti–double-stranded DNA (anti-ds DNA) antibodies are relatively specific for systemic lupus erythematosus (SLE). There are other anti-nuclear antibodies including anti-Sm antibodies that may be noted in the systemic lupus erythematosus (SLE) patient. These are limited in efficacy by both diminished specificity and diminished sensitivity.

E 132 Answer: E

E is correct because hypertension is most unlikely in nephrotic syndrome (NS) due to decreased intravascular volume resulting from the hypoalbuminemia. The hypoalbuminemia is due to the loss of this protein in the urine.

■ You Should Know

1. Nephrotic syndrome (NS) is characterized by proteinuria (>3.5 g/day), hypoalbuminemia, edema, and hyperlipidemia.

2. Nephrotic syndrome (NS) is a glomerular disease that may be due to primary glomerular disease or secondary to a systemic disease.

3. Primary glomerular diseases that may cause nephrotic syndrome (NS) include:
   a. Minimal change disease
   b. Focal segmented glomerulosclerosis
   c. IgA nephropathy

4. Secondary glomerular diseases include:
   a. Diabetes mellitus
   b. Systemic lupus erythematosus
   c. Amyloidosis
   d. HIV nephropathy
   e. Endocarditis

5. Treatment of nephrotic syndrome (NS) includes sodium and fat restriction in the diet, diuretics, angiotensin-converting enzyme inhibitors (ACEI), HMG-CoA reductase inhibitors, and, if needed, heparin/warfarin for deep vein thrombosis.

6. The loss of anti-thrombin in the urine leads to a hypercoagulable state.

7. The hyperlipidemia in nephrotic syndrome (NS) is related to hypercholesterolemia and hypertriglyceridemia that increase risk of cardiovascular disease.

8. Lipid droplets in the urine may be free droplets or within hyaline casts (fatty casts).

E 133   **Answer: B and E**
B is correct because endocarditis is an infection that commonly causes night sweats. E is correct because 25% of Hodgkin's disease patients have night sweats. Less commonly, non-Hodgkin's lymphoma patients have nocturnal sweating.

■ **You Should Know**

1. The infections most commonly associated with night sweats include tuberculosis, symptomatic HIV infection, and endocarditis.

2. Hodgkin's disease has a bimodal age distribution, 20 to 30 years and 50 to 60 years.

3. Medicines are a common cause of night sweats. All anti-depressants, including tricyclics, selective serotonin reuptake inhibitors, and venlafaxine and bupropion can cause night sweats.

4. In addition, medicine-induced hypoglycemia can cause night sweats.

5. Medicines may cause flushing (e.g., niacin, nitroglycerin, tamoxifen, sildenafil and, in susceptible persons, alcohol).

6. The distinction between night sweats and menopausal hot flushes (flashes) may be difficult.

E 134 Answer: A

A is correct because primary (idiopathic) parkinsonism is due to a depletion in the brain of the neurotransmitter dopamine.

■ **You Should Know**

1. Tremor, rigidity, postural instability, and bradykinesia are the primary features of parkinsonism.

2. Parkinsonism is characterized by resting tremor. While typically bilateral, it may be unilateral for a protracted time. The tremor may involve the extremities, lips, and mouth. Gait has small, shuffling steps.

3. Weakness is not characteristic of parkinsonism. Deep tendon reflexes are normal.

4. Medical therapy of parkinsonism includes:
   a. Amantadine
      (1) Best used in mild disease
   b. Anti-cholinergic drugs
      (1) Reduce tremor and rigidity more than bradykinesia; are best in therapy of the younger patient when tremor is the dominant problem
   c. Levodopa or levodopa/carbidopa combination
      (1) Particularly effective in bradykinesia
   d. Dopamine agonists bromocriptine and pergolide
      (1) Ineffective if patient does not respond to levodopa
   e. Monoamine oxidase B inhibitor selegiline
      (1) May slow progression of disease
   f. Catecholamine-O-methyltransferase inhibitors (COMT inhibitors)
      (1) Ineffective when given alone; potentiate the effect of levodopa

5. Adverse effects of levodopa include confusion, hallucinations, agitation, orthostatic hypotension, and involuntary movements.

6. Dopamine agonists and catecholamine-O-methyltransferase inhibitors (COMT) may also cause orthostatic hypotension.

7. Amantadine may cause ankle edema and livedo reticularis.

8. Anti-cholinergic medicines in the elderly may cause memory impairment, confusion, dry mouth, and urinary retention.

9. Essential tremor, which may be familial, is characterized by an intention and postural tremor. (Postural tremor is evident when the patient is holding a weighted object, e.g., a glass of water when the arm is outstretched.) The hands, head, and voice are commonly affected. Otherwise, the neurologic examination is normal. Ingestion of alcohol temporarily suppresses the tremor. Propranolol is the preferred medicinal agent.

E 135 Answer: D

D is correct because fever-associated cytokines, including interleukin, IL-6, and tissue necrosis factor, are produced in tissues and are released by the trauma of surgery. Therefore, fever (i.e., temperature >100.4°F) is common in the first few days after surgery.

You Should Know

1. Postoperative fever may be due to infectious or noninfectious factors.

2. Causes of noninfectious fever, in addition to cytokine release, include:
   a. Medication or blood products—onset of fever is within hours of surgery
   b. Inflammatory conditions (e.g., myocardial infarction, gout, stroke, deep vein thrombosis)

3. Fever whose onset is within the first week of surgery may be related to:
   a. Infection existing before surgery
   b. Pneumonia
   c. Urinary tract infection
   d. Intravascular catheter infection
   e. Occasionally, surgical site infection

4. Fever whose onset is 1 to 4 weeks after surgery may be related to:
   a. Surgical site infection
   b. Febrile reaction to medicines
   c. Noninfectious inflammatory conditions (e.g., myocardial infarction, pulmonary embolism, deep vein thrombosis)

E 136 Answer: B, C, D, and E

C, D, and E are correct because subclavian steal syndrome causes retrograde blood flow in the vertebral artery. The resultant vertebrobasilar artery insufficiency in the brain is associated with symptoms including dizziness, unstable gait, vertigo, diplopia, and bilateral blurred vision. B is correct because the subclavian artery stenosis may result in ischemia of the arm, causing the patient to experience arm claudication or even arm numbness.

You Should Know

1. Subclavian steal syndrome is most commonly due to atherosclerosis and is more common on the left side. In this condition, the subclavian artery is narrowed, resulting in retrograde flow in the ipsilateral vertebral artery.

2. Physical examination shows a significant difference in arm blood pressure, usually >25 mm Hg lower systolic pressure on the affected side.

3. Diagnosis may be made using continuous wave Doppler, duplex ultrasonography, or angiography.

4. Treatment is surgical, either extrathoracic revascularization or percutaneous transluminal angioplasty.

E 137 Answer: E

E is correct because focal glomerulosclerosis is related to heroin nephropathy and heroin nephropathy has a predilection for black patients.

You Should Know

1. Focal glomerulosclerosis (FGS) is an important cause of nephrotic syndrome in children, adolescents, and adults.

2. Focal glomerulosclerosis (FGS) may be primary (idiopathic), which typically presents with acute onset of nephrotic syndrome. Secondary focal glomerulosclerosis (FGS) is related to heroin nephropathy or HIV-associated nephropathy.

E 138   **Answer: A, B and C**
A is correct because maternal smoking during pregnancy increases sudden infant death syndrome (SIDS) risk twofold to fourfold. It may be the most important preventable risk factor. B is correct because low birth weight infants are at a considerably increased risk compared with term infants. C is correct because the incidence of SIDS has dropped significantly since the recommendation that infants be placed in the supine position for sleeping.

■ **You Should Know**

1. SIDS (crib death) is the leading cause of death between 1 month and 1 year of age. SIDS usually occurs between the 2nd and 4th month of age.
2. The cause of SIDS cannot be identified in most cases.

E 139   **Answer: B and E**
B is correct because benign tumors of the liver (adenomas) are more likely to increase in number and size, and more likely to bleed, in women who take oral contraceptives. E is correct because stroke risk is most increased in women who have migraine with aura and who take oral contraceptives.

■ **You Should Know**

1. Oral contraceptives (OC) may be a combination of estrogen and progestin or a progestin minipill.
2. Absolute contraindications to use of a progestin/estrogen oral contraceptives (OC) include:
   a. Pregnancy
   b. Active hepatitis
   c. Thrombogenic mutation (e.g., Factor V Leiden, protein C, protein S, and anti-thrombin deficiency)
   d. Coronary heart disease
   e. History of stroke
   f. Valvular heart disease with pulmonary hypertension, history of endocarditis, or atrial fibrillation
   g. History of deep vein thrombosis or pulmonary embolism
   h. Systolic blood pressure >160 mm Hg
   i. Benign tumor of the liver
   j. Diabetes mellitus with nephropathy or retinopathy
3. Oral contraceptives (OC) may increase the risk of stroke in women who have a history of migraine with aura. Therefore, migraine with aura is considered by some authorities to be an absolute contraindication to oral contraceptives (OC) therapy.

4. Barbiturates, phenytoin, primidone, carbamazepine, and rifampin decrease the efficacy of oral contraceptives (OC).

   5. Benefits of oral contraceptives (OC) include decreased risk of ovarian and endometrial cancer.

E 140   **Answer: A**

A is correct because beta-adrenergic blockers inhibit both gluconeogenesis and glycogenolysis, thus, facilitating hypoglycemia in the patient who takes an antidiabetic medication. In addition, beta blockers may mask the adrenergic manifestations of the low plasma glucose (e.g., sweating, anxiety, and palpitations).

   ■ **You Should Know**

   1. Epinephrine increases glucose production by promoting both glycogenolysis and gluconeogenesis, thus offering protection against the development of hypoglycemia.

   2. Beta-adrenergic blockers slow the resting heart rate and are contraindicated in the patient with sick sinus syndrome unless the patient has an artificial pacemaker.

   3. Beta blockers may increase airway resistance in patients with bronchospastic disease (e.g., asthma). Those blockers with beta-1 selectivity tend to cause a lesser degree of airway impairment.

   4. Beta blockers increase symptoms of claudication in those with moderate to severe arterial occlusive disease. Further, this class of medicine is likely to worsen Raynaud's phenomenon.

E 141   **Answer: D**

D is correct because gestational diabetes screening should be performed between 24 and 28 weeks in women of Native American, African, Hispanic, Pacific Island, and indigenous Australian ancestry.

   ■ **You Should Know**

   1. Gestational screening should also be performed between 24 and 28 weeks in women who are overweight before the pregnancy and in women who have a history of diabetes mellitus in a first-degree relative.

   2. In both diabetic and nondiabetic women fasting glucose levels during pregnancy are lower than during the nonpregnant state.

   3. Exercise lowers plasma glucose concentration by increasing tissue sensitivity to glucose.

   4. In screening the pregnant woman for diabetes, the fasting patient is given an oral 50 g glucose load. Venous plasma glucose concentration is determined 1 hour later. A value of 130 mg/dL or higher indicates a need for a full glucose tolerance test.

   5. In the United States, only insulin is used to treat gestational diabetes. A woman with diabetes who was taking an oral hypoglycemic agent before pregnancy should be converted to insulin therapy during the pregnancy.

E 142   **Answer: B**

B is correct because in the nonpreeclampsia patient, mild hypertension with systolic blood pressure in the 140 to 150 mm Hg range and diastolic pressure in the 90 to 100 mm Hg range is not treated.

You Should Know

1. While there are no strict criteria, it is prudent to initiate antihypertensive therapy in a patient having preeclampsia when systolic blood pressure is 150 mm Hg or higher and diastolic pressure is 100 mm Hg or higher.

2. Labetalol, methyldopa, and long-acting nifedipine are considered effective and safe medications in the pregnant woman. Thiazides appear to play little role overall in the management of hypertension in pregnancy because of the concern over hypovolemia.

3. Angiotensin-converting enzyme inhibitors (ACEI) and angiotensin-receptor blockers are contraindicated in all stages of pregnancy because they are teratogenic. Nitroprusside should be used only as an agent of last resort for intractable, severe hypertension.

4. Beta blockers and calcium channel blockers enter breast milk. Labetalol and propranolol, however, are not concentrated in breast milk.

E 143   **Answer: A, B, C, and D**

A is correct because intravascular hemolysis results in urinary loss of iron in the form of hemosiderinuria and hemoglobinuria. B and C are correct because celiac disease and *Helicobacter pylori* gastritis are associated with decreased gastrointestinal absorption of iron. D is correct because carcinoma of the cecum commonly causes iron deficiency through fecal blood loss.

You Should Know

1. Causes of iron deficiency include:
   a. Blood loss: gastrointestinal bleeding, blood-drawing in medical care, menometrorrhagia
   b. Decreased iron ingestion
   c. Decreased iron absorption: in addition to those previously noted, gastric achlorhydria also is associated with decreased absorption
   d. Intravascular hemolysis

2. Intravascular hemolysis occurs in march hemoglobinuria, defective heart valves, and paroxysmal cold hemoglobinuria.

3. Extravascular hemolysis occurs in the liver, spleen, and bone marrow.

4. Iron stores can be totally depleted while the patient is not anemic. These patients have decreased serum ferritin, the storage iron protein. Yet, these patients will have fatigue and a sense of weakness. Only further depletion of iron will lead to anemia.

5. Increased serum indirect bilirubin, decreased serum haptoglobin, and increased reticulocyte percentage occur in both intravascular and extravascular hemolysis.

6. Iron deficiency is a recognized cause of restless legs syndrome (RLS). Patients have uncomfortable sensations (e.g., creeping, crawling, itching, which occurs only at rest and is relieved immediately by movement). This discomfort is usually bilateral and symptoms characteristically are noted below the knees.

7. The etiology of restless leg syndrome (RLS) include:
   a. Primary, of unknown etiology
   b. Secondary, associated with iron deficiency, pregnancy, end-stage renal disease, diabetes mellitus, and parkinsonism

E 144   **Answer: A and E**
A is correct because alpha-fetoprotein is a maternal serum marker for neural tube defects (NTDs). E is correct because serum alpha-fetoprotein is elevated in 90% of patients who have testicular germ cell tumors.

■ **You Should Know**

1. Neural tube defects (NTDs) are secondary only to cardiac malformations in frequency of congenital anomalies.

2. Two neural tube defects (NTDs) are spina bifida and anencephaly.

3. Neural tube defects (NTDs) risk factors include:
   a. Folic acid deficiency in the mother
   b. Medicines (folate antagonists, valproic acid, and carbamazepine)
   c. Diabetes mellitus
   d. Obesity
   e. Genetic factors

4. All pregnant women should be screened for neural tube defects (NTDs). Alpha-fetoprotein is a maternal serum marker. Maternal screening should be performed at 15 to 20 weeks of gestation.

5. Elevated maternal serum alpha-fetoprotein raises suspicion of neural tube defects (NTDs). An ultrasound and amniocentesis should then be done to assess whether a neural tube defect (NTD) is present.

6. Folic acid supplements reduce the incidence of neural tube defects (NTDs). All pregnant women should ingest daily folic acid supplements. The optimum dosage is not clearly identified. Those women considered to be at higher risk (see earlier) should ingest 4 mg/day during the preconception period and during the pregnancy.

7. Nonpregnant women of reproductive potential should ingest folic acid in a dose of 0.4 to 0.8 mg/day.

8. An increasing serum alpha-fetoprotein level in patients with cirrhosis should raise suspicion of hepatocellular carcinoma.

E 145   **Answer: A**
A is correct because presence of myoglobin or hemoglobin in the urine will cause the dipstick to be positive for blood.

You Should Know

1. A positive dipstick for blood may indicate three different conditions:
   a. Red blood cells in the urine: this will be noted on microscopic urine sediment examination
   b. Hemoglobinuria: no red blood cells will be seen on microscopic exam
   c. Myoglobinuria: as occurs in skeletal muscle breakdown (rhabdomyolysis)

2. Hemoglobinuria occurs in patients who have intravascular hemolysis, as may occur in patients with defective heart valves, march hemoglobinuria, and paroxysmal cold hemoglobinuria.

3. Oral intake of phenazopyridine in treatment of dysuria will cause red/orange discoloration of the urine. The urinary dipstick will not, however, become positive.

E 146   Answer: D

D is correct because parvovirus is the etiologic agent causing fifth disease (erythema infectiosum) that is characterized by a mild febrile illness followed by development of a bilateral malar rash ("slapped cheeks").

You Should Know

1. Children with erythema infectiosum are less likely to have joint manifestations that are common in adults who have parvovirus infection.

2. The clinical manifestation of parvovirus infection depends upon the underlying host. Immunocompetent adults may have no symptoms or may experience a flulike illness followed 1 week later by arthralgia or arthritis.

3. The arthritis or arthralgia is typically symmetrical and involves small joints (e.g., hands, wrists, feet, and knees). Joint symptoms generally resolve in 3 to 4 weeks.

4. Patients with hematologic disease (e.g., sickle cell anemia, iron deficiency anemia) are at increased risk of developing an aplastic crisis with parvovirus infection.

5. Maternal infection with parvovirus during pregnancy can lead to fetal death.

E 147   Answer: D

D is correct because HIV infection typically leads to CD4 T-cell depletion and impaired cellular immunity.

You Should Know

1. HIV type 1 is a human retrovirus that infects lymphocytes and other cells that bear the CD4 surface protein. Ultimately, the immune dysfunction caused by the virus produces clinical AIDS in which opportunistic infections and malignancies arise.

2. The time from initial HIV infection to appearance of clinical AIDS varies from months to years.

3. The virus is transmitted sexually and parenterally.

4. HIV therapy includes:
   a. Anti-retroviral therapy
   b. Prophylaxis of opportunistic infection
   c. Treatment of opportunistic infection
   d. Immunomodulation

5. Anti-retroviral medicines are grouped into four categories:
   a. Nucleoside analog reverse transcriptase inhibitors (NRTIs); examples include didanosine, emtricitabine, stavudine, and zidovudine
   b. Protease inhibitors; examples include indinavir and nelfinavir
   c. Nonnucleoside reverse transcriptase inhibitors; examples include nevirapine and efavirenz
   d. HIV entry inhibitors; an example is enfuvirtide

6. Effective HIV therapy necessitates administration of three or more drugs, often starting with tenofovir, emtricitabine, and efavirenz.

7. Treatment for asymptomatic HIV-infected persons should be initiated when the CD4 cell count is <350 cells/microliter.

8. Zidovudine therapy should be initiated in the HIV-infected pregnant patient, preferably by the 2nd trimester. However, this medicine may be given during labor or delivery and should be given to the newborn.

9. After informed consent where required, HIV serology should be checked in the following:
   a. High-risk persons (e.g., intravenous drug abusers, homosexual and bisexual men, hemophiliacs, sexual partner of known HIV-infected person, prostitutes and their partners, those with sexually transmitted diseases, those who received blood transfusions between 1977 and 1985, and those with multiple sex partners
   b. Pregnant women
   c. Patients with active tuberculosis
   d. Hospitalized patients in communities in which HIV infection is considered to be significant
   e. Donors of blood, semen, and organs
   f. Selected health-care workers and those with occupational exposures

10. Screening for HIV infection is performed with an enzyme-labeled immunosorbent assay (ELISA) for HIV 1 and HIV 2.

11. In the patient with a positive enzyme labeled immunosorbent assay (ELISA), a repeat ELISA is performed in addition to a Western blot. An isolated positive ELISA must be confirmed by a positive Western blot before a definitive diagnosis of HIV infection is made.

12. A person with a positive serology and CD4 lymphocyte count <200 cells/microliter or CD lymphocyte percentage <14% is considered to have AIDS. The CD4 count indicates the amount of HIV immune damage that is already experienced.

13. An HIV-positive patient should have the following tests:
    a. CD4 cell count (normal is 600 to 1500 cells/microliter
    b. Virologic markers including RNA viral load (via polymerase chain reaction); this indicates the magnitude of HIV replication and its associated rate of CD4 cell destruction
    c. Tuberculin skin test

d. Venereal Disease Research Laboratory (VDRL) test
e. Toxoplasma and cytomegalovirus titers
f. Hepatitis A, B (HBsAg, HBsAb, HBcAb), and C serologies
g. *Chlamydia* and gonococcus urine probe

14. HIV-positive persons should receive the following immunizations:
    a. Pneumococcal
    b. Hepatitis A and B
    c. Influenza

E 148   **Answer: D**

D is correct because primary prophylaxis against *Candida* infection appears to promote resistance in *Candida* species.

■ **You Should Know**

1. The use of prophylactic antibiotics has reduced the incidence of opportunistic infection (OI). Prophylaxis for OI includes:
   a. *Pneumocystis carinii* pneumonia for the patient with a CD4 cell count <200 cells/microliter, or CD4 percentage <15%, or unexplained fever lasting longer than 2 weeks, or presence of oral candidiasis. Trimethoprim-sulfamethoxazole (TMP-SMX) is preferred therapy.
   b. Tuberculosis (TBC) prophylaxis in the patient whose tuberculin test shows >5 mm induration or who has had recent contact with a patient known to have active tuberculosis (TBC). Isoniazid (INH) with pyridoxine is preferred.
   c. *Toxoplasma* prophylaxis when CD4 count is <100 cells/microliter. Trimethoprim-sulfamethoxazole (TMP-SMX) or dapsone/pyrimethamine is prescribed.
   d. *Mycobacterium avium* complex prophylaxis is given when the CD4 cell count is <50 cells/microliter. Azithromycin is prescribed.

2. Varicella zoster immune globulin should be given to the patient who has not had chickenpox and who is exposed to a patient with chickenpox or herpes zoster infection (shingles). Zoster vaccination should not be given to an immunocompromised patient.

E 149   **Answer: E**

E is correct because diabetic cranial mononeuropathy most commonly affects cranial nerves III, IV, and VI (the cranial nerves that innervate the extraocular muscles). Further, in 80% of cases of cranial nerve III palsy in the diabetic patient, the pupil size is *normal on the affected side* (in contrast to the usual case of cranial nerve III palsy in which the pupil is enlarged on the affected side).

■ **You Should Know**

1. Diabetic neuropathy includes primarily:
   a. Symmetric polyneuropathy
   b. Cranial nerve mononeuropathy
   c. Peripheral nerve mononeuropathy
   d. Autonomic neuropathy
   e. Diabetic amyotrophy

2. Facial nerve (cranial nerve VII) mononeuropathy, causing Bell's palsy, occurs more frequently in the diabetic patient than in the nondiabetic patient.

3. Symmetrical distal polyneuropathy is the most common type of diabetic neuropathy. This is characterized by progressive sensory loss followed by motor weakness. Patients commonly have burning, tingling and "pins and needles" followed by numbness. Examination shows loss of vibratory sensation, abnormal proprioception, and diminished pain, light touch, and temperature sensation.

4. Peripheral mononeuropathy includes carpal tunnel syndrome, ulnar neuropathy, and peroneal neuropathy, the last causing foot drop.

5. Diabetic amyotrophy is characterized by unilateral thigh pain, weakness, and muscle wasting. Spontaneous recovery occurs in months to years, but may recur on the opposite side.

6. Autonomic neuropathy is considered in E 150.

E 150 Answer: A, B, C, and D
A and C are correct because gastroparesis, characterized by delayed emptying of the stomach, and nocturnal diarrhea are frequent gastrointestinal manifestations of diabetic neuropathy. The etiology of the gastroparesis is multifactorial; nocturnal diarrhea is related to abnormal motility and bacterial overgrowth. B is correct because diabetic neuropathy frequently causes functional disturbance in the sympathetic reflex arc, resulting in the patient having orthostatic hypotension. D is correct because retrograde ejaculation in the diabetic results from impaired sphincter muscle control that is responsible for normal ejaculation.

■ **You Should Know**

1. Poor glycemic control is associated with development of diabetic autonomic neuropathy (DAN). Obversely, vigorous control of plasma glucose slows onset and slows progression of DAN.

2. Diabetic autonomic neuropathy (DAN) involves both the sympathetic and parasympathetic divisions of the autonomic nervous system.

3. Diabetic autonomic neuropathy (DAN) affects different organ systems:
    a. Cardiovascular
    b. Genitourinary
    c. Gastrointestinal
    d. Sudomotor (sweating)
    e. Ophthalmic
    f. Neuroendocrine

4. Cardiovascular manifestations of diabetic autonomic neuropathy (DAN) include:
    a. Orthostatic hypotension: diabetic autonomic neuropathy (DAN)-induced orthostatic hypotension is not characterized by a compensatory heart rate increase as the blood pressure drops, in contrast to hypovolemia-induced orthostatic hypotension in which heart rate increases as pressure falls
    b. Lack of variation in heart rate, which is considered to be a risk factor for sudden cardiac death

5. Gastroparesis is manifest by anorexia, nausea, vomiting, and wide swings in plasma glucose concentration despite vigorous patient efforts.

6. Genitourinary manifestations of diabetic autonomic neuropathy (DAN) include:
   a. Retrograde ejaculation, often manifest as cloudy urine after intercourse
   b. Erectile dysfunction
   c. Dyspareunia related to decreased vaginal lubrication
   d. Overflow incontinence of urine due to the patient's inability to sense a full bladder

7. Patients with diabetic autonomic neuropathy (DAN) may have distal anhidrosis (lack of sweating) with central hyperhidrosis.

8. Diabetic autonomic neuropathy (DAN) patients may have decreased glucagon and epinephrine secretion in response to hypoglycemia.

E 151   Answer: D

D is correct because placenta previa, typically, is characterized by 3rd trimester bleeding that is painless because there are no associated uterine contractions.

■ **You Should Know**

1. 1st trimester vaginal bleeding occurs in ~30% of pregnant women.

2. The three major causes of *1st trimester bleeding* are:
   a. Ectopic pregnancy
   b. Threatened or imminent abortion
   c. Disease of the cervix, uterus, or vagina

3. In the patient having bleeding in the 1st trimester, passage of blood clots, passage of tissue, or pelvic cramping make ectopic pregnancy and miscarriage more likely.

4. Two or more consecutive pregnancy losses after 10 weeks of gestation suggest anti-phospholipid antibody syndrome.

5. After physical examination, ultrasonography is the preferred diagnostic test for evaluation of bleeding during early pregnancy.

6. The most common causes of *3rd trimester bleeding* include:
   a. Placenta previa
   b. Abruptio placentae

7. Digital exam should not be performed in the patient presenting with late bleeding until placenta previa has been excluded.

8. Risk factors for placenta previa include multiple cesarean sections and multiparity.

9. Clinically, abruption placenta presents with vaginal bleeding, uterine contractions, and abdominal tenderness.

10. Risk factors for abruptio placentae include hypertension, smoking, cocaine use, prior abruptio placentae, advanced maternal age, and uterine fibroids.

11. Ultrasonography rarely shows abruption but is important to exclude placenta previa.

E 152 **Answer: D**

D is correct because the post-splenectomy patient is at risk for sepsis caused by encapsulated bacteria (e.g., *Haemophilus influenza*, *Streptococcus pneumoniae*, and *Neisseria meningitidis*).

■ **You Should Know**

1. The spleen is the primary site for production of IgM antibodies that opsonize encapsulated bacteria.

2. At least 2 weeks before elective splenectomy the patient should receive pneumococcal vaccine, *Haemophilus* B conjugate vaccine, and meningococcal vaccine.

3. Children who have undergone splenectomy or those with impaired splenic function (e.g., sickle cell anemia), should take daily penicillin for at least 3 to 5 years or until adulthood.

E 153 **Answer: A, B, and C**

A and C are correct because both hypovolemia and gastrointestinal (GI) bleeding reduce oxygen delivery to the liver. Further, degradation of blood products in gastrointestinal (GI) bleeding leads to increased ammonia delivery to the liver. B is correct because hypokalemia leads to intracellular acidosis which, in turn, results in increased production of ammonia.

■ **You Should Know**

1. The diagnosis of hepatic encephalopathy (HE) is not based upon blood ammonia concentration.

2. Hepatic encephalopathy (HE) typically occurs in patients who have advanced chronic liver disease with signs including jaundice, ascites, palmar erythema, spider telangiectasia, and muscle wasting. Since the patient with chronic liver disease and ascites is not in right heart failure, the central (jugular) venous pressure (CVP) is normal. However, in the unusual case when the ascites is very tense, the central (jugular) venous pressure (CVP) may be elevated. In this case, paracentesis will cause the central (jugular) venous pressure (CVP) to quickly decrease to normal levels.

3. Other precipitating causes of hepatic encephalopathy (HE) include:
   a. Hypoxemia
   b. Sedatives/ tranquilizers

4. Treatment of hepatic encephalopathy (HE) includes oral or rectal lactulose, dietary protein restriction and oral neomycin. The lactulose increases ammonium excretion in the stool, and modifies colonic bacterial flora. Neomycin reduces the number of ammonia-producing bacteria in the bowel.

5. Treatment of ascites associated with cirrhosis usually includes a combination of spironolactone and furosemide.

E 154 **Answer: C and E**

C is correct because the decreased glomerular filtration rate in advanced renal disease results in hyperphosphatemia. E is correct because the decreased renal production of erythropoietin in advanced renal disease leads to a normochromic normocytic anemia.

■ You Should Know

1. Chronic renal disease is characterized by hyperkalemia, hypocalcemia, hyperphosphatemia, and metabolic acidosis.

2. Complications of chronic renal disease include:
   a. Cardiovascular:
      (1) Hypertension
      (2) Pericarditis
      (3) Heart failure
   b. Neurologic:
      (1) Encephalopathy manifest by confusion, lethargy, and coma. Signs include hyperreflexia, asterixis, and nystagmus
      (2) Neuropathy manifest by stocking glove sensorimotor polyneuropathy with loss of deep tendon reflexes
   c. Mineral metabolism
      (1) Osteitis fibrosa cystica from secondary hyperparathyroidism
      (2) Osteomalacia
   d. Skin
      (1) Pruritus

E 155   Answer: E

E is correct because the low cardiac output and reduced arterial pressure associated with systolic heart failure leads to increased secretion of anti-diuretic hormone (ADH). Increased anti-diuretic hormone (ADH) secretion causes hyponatremia.

■ You Should Know

1. The hyponatremia (serum sodium <135 mEq/L) patient may be asymptomatic in mild cases. In more severe cases, nausea, vomiting, weakness, confusion, stupor, seizure, and coma may be present.

2. Hyponatremia is categorized by:
   a. Serum osmolality (normal: 280 to 285 mOsm/kg)
   b. Extracellular fluid (ECF) volume

3. Serum osmolality determination enables hyponatremia to be categorized by:
   a. Isotonic hyponatremia
   b. Hypertonic hyponatremia
   c. Hypotonic hyponatremia

4. Isotonic hyponatremia is usually caused by marked elevation in serum proteins or lipids (e.g., triglycerides or chylomicrons).

5. Hypertonic hyponatremia is most commonly due to marked hyperglycemia.

6. Hypotonic hyponatremia is divided by extracellular volume into three categories:
   a. Volume depletion, with orthostatic hypotension and poor turgor
   b. Volume expansion, with peripheral edema
   c. Euvolemia (normal extracellular fluid [ECF] volume)

7. Volume depletion hyponatremia occurs in cases of excessive nonrenal losses of sodium and water, replaced by excess water alone or water with inadequate salt intake (as might occur in a long-distance runner) or by adrenal insufficiency.

8. Euvolemic hyponatremia occurs typically in syndrome of inappropriate anti-diuretic hormone secretion (SIADH) that may occur in central nervous system tumor or infection, malignancy (small cell carcinoma of lung, carcinoma of pancreas, lymphoma) or due to medicines (e.g., tricyclic antidepressants, cyclophosphamide, thiothixene, carbamazepine).

9. Increased volume hyponatremia occurs in:
   a. Heart failure
   b. Cirrhosis with ascites
   c. Nephrotic syndrome

E 156   **Answer: A, B, D, and E**
A, B, and D are correct because hyponatremia, hypocalcemia, and uremia are brain *nonstructural* causes of seizures. E is correct because encephalitis is a *structural* (i.e., inflammatory), brain disorder that may be associated with seizures.

■ **You Should Know**

1. Other causes of nonstructural seizures include:
   a. Acute withdrawal of drugs (e.g., benzodiazepines)
   b. Drug intoxication (e.g., cocaine, methamphetamine)
   c. Medicine effects (e.g., cyclosporine, imipenem)
   d. Epilepsy

2. Other causes of structural seizures include:
   a. Primary or metastatic brain tumor
   b. Brain infections (e.g., meningitis)
   c. Brain trauma or hemorrhage
   d. Cerebrovascular accident

3. Transient ischemic attacks (TIAs) last minutes to hours. They generally are associated with "negative" manifestations (e.g., weakness, visual loss, or numbness).

4. In contrast, seizures are associated with "positive" neurologic symptoms and signs (e.g., jerking, stiffness or visual hallucinations).

5. Encephalitis should be suspected in the patient who has fever and neurologic signs, especially personality change, motor or sensory deficits, seizures, but without meningeal signs. Herpes simplex virus is the most common cause of encephalitis.

6. In contrast to encephalitis, patients with meningitis tend to have intact cerebral function.

E 157   **Answer: E**
E is correct because dehydration occurs when there is a lack of replacement of usual or increased body water loss. The water loss leads to hypernatremia, an increase in plasma sodium concentration.

You Should Know

1. Hypernatremia is caused by:
    a. Dehydration
    b. Renal loss of water
        (1) Central diabetes insipidus (involvement of the pituitary or hypothalamus by tumor, trauma, infection, or stroke)
        (2) Nephrogenic diabetes insipidus (genetic or related to therapy with lithium or Declomycin)
        (3) Osmotic diuresis (related to glycosuria or tube feedings)
    c. Extrarenal (sweating, burns)
    d. Increased sodium intake (hypertonic saline)

E 158 Answer: A, B, and C

A is correct because sweating is an *autonomic* (adrenergic) manifestation of hypoglycemia. B and C are correct because confusion and seizures are *neuroglycopenic* manifestations of hypoglycemia.

You Should Know

1. Hypoglycemia most commonly occurs in the diabetic population due to inappropriate glycemic therapy, either insulin or oral preparations.

2. Hypoglycemic symptoms are either autonomic or neuroglycopenic.

3. Autonomic symptoms include:
    a. Tremulousness
    b. Sweating
    c. Palpitations
    d. Hunger
    e. Tingling sensation

4. Neuroglycopenic manifestations include:
    a. Impaired concentration
    b. Confusion
    c. Seizures
    d. Coma

5. Important clinical point: hypoglycemia may cause *localized neurologic signs* (e.g., hemiplegia).

6. Fasting hypoglycemia may be due to:
    a. Insulinoma, an insulin-secreting tumor
    b. Alcohol abuse
    c. Advanced hepatic or renal disease
    d. Glucocorticoid deficit (adrenal or pituitary insufficiency)

7. Postprandial hypoglycemia may be due to:
    a. Bariatric surgery or other gastric/intestinal surgery
    b. Functional hypoglycemia (an imprecise term related to patients who have symptoms 3 to 5 hours after meals. In these patients there is no clear correlation between symptoms and plasma glucose levels.)

8. Hypoglycemia associated with alcohol intake may be related to decreased food intake, reduced hepatic glycogen storage, or deficiency of the enzyme

that metabolizes alcohol. Hypoglycemia, manifest by coma or seizures, may occur with binge alcohol drinking and can be mistaken for alcohol intoxication or withdrawal.

9. Dumping syndrome should not be confused with hypoglycemia, though the symptoms are similar. Symptoms occur within 1 hour of eating and may be related to contraction of plasma volume due to fluid shifts into the bowel.

E 159 **Answer: A, D and E**

A is correct because carcinoma of the cervix is an anogenital malignancy related to human papillomavirus (HPV) infection. D is correct because condylomata acuminata, due to human papillomavirus (HPV) infection, is an anogenital cutaneous lesion and is the most common viral, sexually transmitted disease in the United States. E is correct because another cutaneous manifestation of human papillomavirus (HPV) infection is plantar warts.

You Should Know

1. HPV infection most commonly causes cutaneous and anogenital diseases.

2. Cutaneous manifestations of human papillomavirus (HPV) infection include:
   a. Common warts (verruca vulgaris)
   b. Plantar warts
   c. Flat (juvenile) warts

3. Anogenital manifestations of human papillomavirus (HPV) infection include:
   a. Condylomata acuminata
   b. Carcinoma of the cervix, anus, vulva, penis, and vagina

4. Cervical infection by human papillomavirus (HPV) is associated with virtually all cases of cervical cancer.

5. Laboratory diagnosis of human papillomavirus (HPV) infection include:
   a. Cytology (Papanicolaou smear)
   b. Molecular-based methods, including human papillomavirus (HPV) DNA testing in selected patients

6. Immunization with human papillomavirus (HPV) vaccine is recommended in females 9 to 26 years of age.

E 160 **Answer: A**

A is correct because delirium tremens in the patient with a history of sustained alcohol intake characteristically starts with 48 to 96 hours of abstinence. Hallucinations, disorientation, low-grade fever, agitation, and diaphoresis are common manifestations.

You Should Know

1. Alcohol withdrawal syndromes include:
   a. Minor withdrawal
   b. Withdrawal seizures
   c. Alcoholic hallucinosis
   d. Delirium tremens

2. Minor withdrawal usually occurs 5 to 30 hours after the last drink and is manifest by insomnia, tremulousness, headache, and sweating.

3. Withdrawal seizures are generalized tonic-clonic convulsions that usually occur 6 to 48 hours after the last drink.

4. Alcoholic hallucinosis, occurring typically 12 to 48 hours after the last drink, is characterized most frequently by visual hallucinations, though auditory or tactile hallucinations may occur. The sensorium is not clouded.

5. Thiamine, either intramuscularly or intravenously, should promptly be given to all patients with alcohol withdrawal symptoms or signs.

6. Benzodiazepines are the first-line agents for all alcohol withdrawal clinical syndromes.

E 161   Answer: A

A is correct because the typical presentation of infantile hypertrophic pyloric stenosis (IHPS) is a 3-to-6-week-old baby who has immediate postprandial, nonbilious vomiting.

■ **You Should Know**

1. Infantile hypertrophic pyloric stenosis (IHPS) is 4-to-6 times more common in male infants.

2. Neonatal administration of a macrolide antibiotic appears to increase the incidence of infantile hypertrophic pyloric stenosis (IHPS).

3. Ultrasound or upper gastrointestinal contrast study can be used for diagnosis.

4. Definitive therapy is surgical.

E 162   Answer: C

C is correct because the patient whose plasma glucose cannot be controlled with metformin requires therapy with a second medicine that has a different mechanism of action in lowering the glucose levels. It is common to use a sulfonylurea in addition to the metformin.

■ **You Should Know**

1. Two fasting plasma glucose values >126 mg/dL suggests diabetes mellitus. A random glucose level, the least acceptable test for diagnosis, >200 mg/dL, in the presence of diabetic symptoms, indicates diabetes mellitus. A 2-hour glucose tolerance test value >200 mg/dL is diagnostic.

2. In the patient with type 2 diabetes, an HbA1c value less than 7% is considered optimum control.

3. Rigorous glycemic control reduces the risk of microvascular diabetic complications.

4. Biguanides (e.g., metformin), suppress hepatic glucose production, decrease intestinal absorption of glucose, and improve insulin sensitivity.

5. Sulfonylureas increase pancreatic secretion of insulin.

6. Thiazolidinediones (e.g., rosiglitazone and pioglitazone) increase sensitivity to insulin.

7. Alpha-glucosidase inhibitors (e.g., acarbose and miglitol) reduce gastrointestinal absorption of carbohydrate.

8. Meglitinides (e.g., repaglinide and nateglinide) increase pancreatic secretion of insulin.

9. Urine glucose testing is not recommended because it does not adequately assess glycemic status.

E 163   **Answer: E**

E is correct because the Aviation Medical Assistance Act of 1998 states that legal immunity from malpractice litigation is, in part, based upon the Samaritan not receiving compensation for the medical intervention. Seat upgrades and travel vouchers do not count as compensation.

■ **You Should Know**

1. The Aviation Medical Assistance Act of 1998 offers legal protection against malpractice litigation if the following conditions are met:
   a. Samaritan is medically qualified to perform service
   b. Samaritan acts voluntarily
   c. Samaritan acts in good faith
   d. Samaritan does not engage in gross negligence
   e. Samaritan receives no compensation

2. The aircraft cabin environment during flight is characterized by:
   a. Reduced oxygen pressure
   b. Pressurization to 5000 to 8000 feet above sea level
   c. Low humidity (10% to 20%)
   d. Ventilation system maintains low bacteria and fungi counts
   e. Significant vibration

3. The low humidity can trigger medical problems, especially in patients with asthma and chronic obstructive lung disease, due to drying of mucus in the bronchial airways.

E 164   **Answer: D and E**

D is correct because intravenous immune globulin is highly effective in raising the platelet count in idiopathic thrombocytopenic purpura (ITP), but its effect lasts only 1 to 2 weeks. E is correct because immune globulin plus aspirin reduces the risk of coronary artery aneurysm in Kawasaki disease patients.

■ **You Should Know**

1. Therapy of idiopathic thrombocytopenic purpura (ITP) includes a glucocorticoid, typically prednisone, in a tapering course over 4 to 6 weeks after the platelet count has returned to normal.

2. Intravenous immune globulin administration in the idiopathic thrombocytopenic purpura (ITP) is reserved for cases of bleeding emergencies and, at times, preparing a patient for surgery.

3. Kawasaki disease, a vasculitis of immune etiology, is characterized by fever, conjunctivitis, erythema of lips and oral mucosa, "strawberry" tongue, and adenopathy. The major complication is coronary artery aneurysm formation that may lead to acute myocardial infarction, arrhythmia, and sudden cardiac death.

E 165   **Answer: B**
B is correct because spider angiomata result from alterations in sex hormone metabolism that occur in chronic liver disease. The increase in estradiol/free testosterone ratio is thought related to the development of these vascular lesions that have a central arteriole surrounded by smaller vessels.

■ **You Should Know**

1. Stigmata of hepatic cirrhosis include:
   a. Palmar erythema
   b. Abdominal wall collateral veins (caput medusae)
   c. Gynecomastia
   d. Ascites
   e. Dupuytren's contracture
   f. Jaundice
   g. Testicular atrophy
   h. Peripheral neuropathy (sensory or sensorimotor—not autonomic)
   i. Esophageal and gastric varices due to portal hypertension

E 166   **Answer: A, B and C**
A is correct because oral contraceptives (OCs) increase serum triglyceride concentration. B is correct because oral contraceptives (OCs) can worsen liver function in patients who have active liver disease. C is correct because oral contraceptives (OCs) increase risk of thrombosis in women who have a history of thrombosis (e.g., stroke or deep vein thrombosis).

■ **You Should Know**

1. Oral contraceptives (OCs) increase the risk of thrombosis in women >35 years of age who smoke 15 or more cigarettes per day or those women who have a history of thrombosis.

2. Before initiating oral contraceptive (OC) therapy, determine whether concomitant medicinal intake by the patient could influence the efficacy of the oral contraceptives (OCs). Phenytoin, rifampin, and St. John's wort decrease oral contraceptive (OC) effectiveness.

3. Oral contraceptives (OCs) reduce the risk of ovarian cancer.

4. Oral contraceptives (OCs) may increase the risk of stroke in women who have a history of migraine with aura. Therefore, migraine with aura is considered by many to be an absolute contraindication to oral contraceptive (OC) therapy.

E 167   **Answer: A, B, C, and D**

A is correct because polycystic ovary syndrome is associated with increased insulin resistance. Therefore, diabetes mellitus is common. B is correct because hypercortisolism increases insulin resistance and, thus, causes hyperglycemia. C is correct because growth hormone antagonizes the action of insulin, thus causing hyperglycemia. D is correct because the increased catecholamine secretion in pheochromocytoma promotes gluconeogenesis and glycogenolysis and induces tissue resistance to insulin.

You Should Know

1. Polycystic ovary syndrome is characterized by infertility, obesity, hirsutism, and oligomenorrhea (or amenorrhea). Abnormal laboratory values include high testosterone, estrogen, and luteinizing hormone levels in the serum. Insulin resistance and diabetes mellitus are common.

2. Hypercortisolism, due to pituitary adenoma (Cushing's disease), adrenal hyperplasia or carcinoma, or exogenous glucocorticoid therapy all are associated with hyperglycemia due to insulin resistance. These patients often have hypertension, truncal obesity, ecchymoses, rounded face (moon facies), and psychological manifestations that may include euphoria, depression, and even psychosis.

3. Acromegaly results from excess growth hormone secretion by a pituitary adenoma. It is characterized by enlargement of the hands, feet and jaw, coarsening of facial features, hypertension (50%), and diabetes mellitus (30%). The adenoma secretes both growth hormone and prolactin.

4. Pheochromocytomas are tumors that secrete excessive quantities of norepinephrine and epinephrine. Most have sustained hypertension (a smaller percentage having paroxysmal hypertension). Episodic sweats, headache, and palpitation lasting minutes to hours are characteristic. Diagnosis is established in most cases by assay of urinary catecholamines and metanephrines. Only pheochromocytoma is associated with hypertension and orthostatic hypotension.

5. In the patient who has hypertension and hyperglycemia, think of the following:
   a. Pheochromocytoma
   b. Hypercortisolism
   c. Acromegaly
   d. The diabetic patient who develops hypertension secondary to progressive renal involvement

6. Medullary carcinoma of the thyroid may produce one or more chemicals, including calcitonin, serotonin, prostaglandin, and adrenocorticotrophic hormone. Flushing and diarrhea may be presenting symptoms.

E 168   **Answer: D**

D is correct because nonaspirin, nonselective, nonsteroidal anti-inflammatory agents (NSAIDs) inhibit renal vasodilator prostaglandins. As a result, blood pressure increases.

■ You Should Know

1. Nonaspirin, nonsteroidal anti-inflammatory medicines (NSAIDS) increase salt and water reabsorption in the kidney. Thus, a normal person will gain 0.5 to 1 kg in weight. Those with cirrhosis or heart failure may gain much more weight due to exaggerated salt and water retention.

2. Adverse effects of NSAIDS include:
   a. Rash, localized hyperpigmentation or bullae
   b. Edema
   c. Peptic ulcer
   d. Prerenal failure, especially in the hypovolemic patient
   e. Hyperkalemia, most commonly in the patient who takes the NSAID in conjunction with an angiotensin-converting enzyme inhibitor (ACEI) or the chronic renal disease patient who takes an NSAID
   f. Colitis
   g. Post-surgical oozing, due to the anti-platelet effect of NSAIDS that is similar to that of aspirin

3. Phosphodiesterase-5 inhibitors (e.g., sildenafil, vardenafil, and tadalafil), can cause profound hypotension when taken in conjunction with a nitrates. This class of medicine must be used with caution in men who take alpha-adrenergic blockers.

E 169   Answer: A and B

A and B are correct because trichinellosis and ascariasis are parasitic diseases that invade tissue. The tissue invasion elicits an immune response resulting in eosinophilia. Eosinophiles attack parasites, but not bacteria.

■ You Should Know

1. Trichinellosis is caused by the parasite *Trichinella* and is often related to ingestion of uncooked meat. Initial symptoms may be nausea, vomiting, and diarrhea or the patient may be asymptomatic until skeletal muscles are invaded.

2. In trichinellosis, skeletal muscle pain is typical, often associated with fever. Splinter hemorrhages, periorbital edema, and conjunctival hemorrhages occur at this time

3. *Ascaris lumbricoides*, a roundworm, causes varied clinical manifestations, including:
   a. Pulmonary involvement, with pneumonia
   b. Intestinal involvement, with nausea, vomiting, and diarrhea. However, in children between ages 1 and 5 years, intestinal obstruction is common

4. Systemic lupus erythematosus (SLE) is typically associated with leukopenia, thrombocytopenia, and, occasionally, hemolytic anemia. Some systemic lupus erythematosus (SLE) patients have anti-phospholipid antibodies that increase the risk of venous and arterial thrombosis.

E 170   Answer: A, C and E

A is correct because hypertension is the most important predisposing cause of dissection. C is correct because the abrupt, transient increase in blood pressure associated with crack cocaine use results in an intimal tear in the aorta with attendant dissection. E is correct because Marfan' syndrome, an inherited disorder of connective tissue, causes weakening of the aorta media, thus predisposing to dissection.

You Should Know

1. Aortic dissection begins with an intimal tear followed by development of a dissecting hematoma in the media of the aorta wall.

2. Adult patients most commonly have the dissection in the 5th through 7th decades. In this group, hypertension is the most common predisposing factor.

3. Younger patients with dissection generally have a congenital anomaly or inherited defect in connective tissue.

4. Congenital anomalies associated with dissection include:
   a. Coarctation of aorta
   b. Bicuspid aortic valve

5. Connective tissue disorders associated with dissection include:
   a. Marfan's syndrome
   b. Ehlers-Danlos syndrome

E 171 Answer: A

A is correct because central vertigo is associated with other neurologic symptoms and signs including diplopia, ataxia, visual loss, slurred speech, weakness, and numbness. Physical examination may show dysmetria and abnormal reflexes.

You Should Know

1. Dizziness is nonspecific and may refer to vertigo, presyncope, and disequilibrium.

2. Vertigo is a sensation of movement. It can be related to peripheral or central vestibular dysfunction.

3. The peripheral system refers to the inner ear; the central to the brainstem and cerebellum.

4. Benign positional vertigo and Ménière's disease are peripheral causes of vertigo. Vertebrobasilar artery insufficiency, brain stem infarction, and cerebellar infarction are central causes.

5. Peripheral vertigo is typically not associated with other neurologic symptoms.

6. Nausea and vomiting can occur with both central and peripheral vertigo.

7. Nystagmus may be noted in patients having both central and peripheral vertigo.

8. A patient with vertigo who also has tinnitus suggests a peripheral origin of the vertigo.

9. Presyncope refers to "almost blacking out" from cerebral hypoperfusion. This may occur with orthostatic hypotension or cardiac arrhythmia.

10. Disequilibrium is imbalance in walking. Peripheral neuropathy, cervical spondylosis, and muscular diseases may cause gait instability.

E 172 Answer: E

E is correct because carbon monoxide binds with the iron in hemoglobin resulting in formation of carboxyhemoglobin. Pulse oximetry cannot screen for carbon monoxide poisoning because oximetry cannot differentiate between oxyhemoglobin and carboxyhemoglobin.

You Should Know

1. Carbon monoxide (CO) is colorless, odorless, and tasteless.

2. Smoke inhalation is the most common cause of carbon monoxide (CO) poisoning (e.g., exposure) to a poorly ventilated, fuel-burning heater or a poorly functioning heating system.

3. Headache is the most common presenting system. Nausea and dizziness followed by change in mental status (confusion to coma) may follow.

4. Systemic arterial pO2 (Pa_{O_2}) is usually *normal* in carbon monoxide (CO) poisoning because pO2 (P_{O_2}) reflects oxygen that is dissolved in blood.

5. The "cherry red" skin sign in carbon monoxide (CO) poisoning is very insensitive.

6. Carbon monoxide (CO) poisoning is treated with high-flow, face mask oxygen inhalation.

E 173 Answer: E

E is correct because the cremasteric reflex is typically present in the patient who has torsion of the appendix testis but is absent in the patient who has testicular torsion.

You Should Know

1. The differential diagnosis of acute scrotal pain in children and adolescents includes:
   a. Testicular torsion
   b. Torsion of appendix testis
   c. Epididymitis
   d. Orchitis
   e. Henoch-Schönlein purpura
   f. Inguinal hernia

2. Color Doppler ultrasonography is the preferred diagnostic test used to differentiate amongst these conditions.

3. Testicular torsion is occasionally seen in neonates, but most commonly occurs in post-pubertal boys (though it can occur at any age). Pain is sudden in onset and often occurs several hours after strenuous physical activity. Physical examination shows an exquisitely tender testis, high-riding testis on the affected side, with the long axis of the testis oriented transversely ("bell-clapper deformity"). The cremasteric reflex is usually absent. Immediate surgical intervention is necessary.

4. The onset of pain is usually more gradual in torsion of the appendix testis. This is the most common cause of acute scrotal pain. Eighty percent (80%) of cases occur between the ages of 7 and 14 years. Inspection of the scrotal wall may show a "blue dot" sign representing infarction of the appendix testis.

Treatment may be conservative (e.g., a nonsteroidal anti-inflammatory [NSAIDs] medicine) or surgical.

5. Epididymitis may be acute, but also occurs in a subacute form. *Acute* epididymitis is characterized by severe pain and swelling, usually associated with fever, chills, and voiding symptoms. Physical examination shows induration, swelling, and exquisite tenderness of the involved epididymis. In the sexually active male, *Chlamydia* is the most common infecting organism though gonococcus, and other organisms may be causative.

6. Orchitis may be caused by multiple viruses (e.g., mumps, coxsackie, and others). It is characterized by scrotal swelling and shininess of the skin, and tenderness of the testis.

7. *Subacute* epididymitis usually occurs in healthy men related to sexual activity, heavy physical exertion, or bicycle/motorcycle riding.

E 174   **Answer: A and E**

A is correct because a headache that starts suddenly and reaches maximum intensity within seconds is suggestive of subarachnoid hemorrhage (SAH). E is correct because a headache that starts with exertion (e.g., walking or Valsalva strain), suggests intracranial hemorrhage, carotid artery dissection, or pheochromocytoma.

■ **You Should Know**

1. The clinician must differentiate life-threatening headache (e.g., meningitis, subarachnoid hemorrhage [SAH], brain tumor), from benign headache (e.g., cluster, migraine, and tension).

2. Patients who have subarachnoid hemorrhage (SAH) typically have sudden onset of the headache with nausea and vomiting. This is followed very quickly, in many cases, by seizures and loss of consciousness. Subarachnoid hemorrhages (SAHs) are due to rupture of cerebral aneurysms, cocaine/amphetamine abuse, and arteriovenous malformations.

3. Cluster headache is always unilateral. It is deep and excruciating in the area of the eye or temple. The headache is accompanied by autonomic signs (e.g., tearing, nasal congestion, and Horner's syndrome). Alcohol is a common precipitating factor.

E 175   **Answer: B**

B is correct because uncomplicated cystitis in the healthy, nonpregnant woman is treated with 3 days of a fluoroquinolone, or 7 days of nitrofurantoin, or 3 days of trimethoprim-sulfamethoxazole (TMP-SMX). TMP-SMX, however, appears now to have a significant number of resistant organisms.

■ **You Should Know**

1. Dysuria in women, manifest by pain or burning upon urination, is caused by inflammation of the urethra, bladder, or vagina. The inflammation may or may not be related to infection.

2. Common infectious causes of dysuria include bacterial cystitis, chlamydial urethritis, acute pyelonephritis, gonococcal urethritis, *Trichomonas* urethritis,

and vaginitis. Vaginal itching or discharge significantly reduces the likelihood of cystitis.

3. Pyuria is almost always noted in the patient who has bacterial cystitis, pyelonephritis, and chlamydial or gonococcal urethritis. Pyuria is not typically present in the woman with vaginitis. The presence of hematuria effectively rules out vaginitis.

4. The urinalysis is the most important diagnostic test in the healthy, young, nonpregnant woman with dysuria. Pyuria with bacteriuria is found in bacterial cystitis, most commonly due to *Escherichia coli, Staphylococcus saprophyticus,* and enterococci. Urine culture and sensitivity should be reserved for those suspected of having a complicated urinary tract infection.

5. Complicated urinary infections occur in those who:
   a. Have diabetes mellitus
   b. Have a history of childhood urinary tract infections
   c. Have had three urinary tract infections in the past year
   d. Have an indwelling urethral catheter
   e. Have a hospital-acquired urinary infection

6. The examination of the urine in the patient with chlamydial urethritis shows pyuria but no bacteria. No blood is noted. The ligase chain reaction test appears to be the best diagnostic test. The nonpregnant patient is treated with azithromycin or doxycycline.

7. In addition to dysuria, the woman with a gonococcal infection may have a purulent urethral discharge. Urinalysis shows pyuria without bacteriuria, but Gram stain of the urethral discharge shows gram-negative diplococci. Ceftriaxone or cefpodoxime is the preferred therapy. Sex partners should be treated. Patients should be empirically treated for *Chlamydia*.

8. Bacterial vaginosis (BV) is the most common cause of vaginitis in women of childbearing age. It is due to an increase in the number of many organisms, most notably, *Gardnerella*. The patient frequently has a "fishy smelling" thin vaginal discharge. Diagnosis is based upon a positive whiff-amine test, defined as a fishy odor when 10% potassium hydroxide is added to vaginal discharge specimens. Clue cells, vaginal epithelial cells with adherent coccobacilli, are the most reliable predictor of bacterial vaginosis (BV). Oral metronidazole or intravaginal clindamycin is an effective therapy.

9. *Trichomonas vaginalis* may be an asymptomatic condition, but classically, causes vaginal burning and pruritus, dysuria, and a malodorous, thin vaginal discharge. Examination shows a "strawberry" cervix (i.e., punctate hemorrhages on the cervix) and a green-yellow frothy discharge. Wet mount preparations show motile trichomonads. Therapy of the nonpregnant patient is metronidazole. Sexual partners should be treated.

10. Patients with chlamydial or gonococcal urethritis should be tested for HIV infection and syphilis.

E 176   Answer: E

E is correct because *Escherichia coli* and *Pseudomonas* are the two most common organisms causing acute bacterial prostatitis.

You Should Know

1. Acute bacterial prostatitis is characterized by fever, chills, dysuria, and discomfort, often in the low back and perineum. *Escherichia coli* and *Pseudomonas* are the most common infecting organisms, but less frequently, the gram-positive enterococci are the infecting agents. The patient may require hospitalization for parenteral therapy (ampicillin plus aminoglycoside until infecting organism is defined on culture) followed by a therapeutic regimen lasting 4 to 6 weeks. Gram-negative rods are treated with quinolones or trimethoprim-sulfamethoxazole. (TMX-SMX). Gram-positive enterococci are treated with ampicillin or amoxicillin. After completion of antibiotic therapy, urine culture and sensitivity and prostatic secretion examination should be performed.

2. Chronic bacterial prostatitis may be related to both gram-negative and gram-positive organisms. Patients commonly have dysuria and frequency. Analysis of the urine is frequently normal. Prostatic secretion analysis shows increased number of leukocytes (>10/high-power field). Diagnosis is based upon culture of prostatic secretions or post-massage urine specimen. Trimethoprim-sulfamethoxazole (TMX-SMX) or quinolones are administered for 4 to 12 weeks.

3. Nonbacterial prostatitis is common and is of unknown etiology. Patients have dysuria and discomfort in the perineal and suprapubic areas. Prostatic secretions show an increased number of leukocytes, but all cultures are sterile. There is no completely effective therapy.

E 177 **Answer: E**

E is correct because absence of ankle deep tendon reflexes is noted in 50% of persons between the ages of 81 and 90 years who have no recognized nervous system disease.

You Should Know

1. Horner's syndrome is characterized by miosis, ptosis, and facial anhidrosis. It may arise from lesions in the brainstem and cervical/thoracic spinal cord in which sympathetic fibers are disrupted. Causes of Horner's syndrome include:
   a. Bronchogenic carcinoma with spread into the inferior sympathetic ganglion
   b. Cluster headache
   c. Cerebellar infarction due to thrombosis of inferior cerebellar artery
   d. Dissection of carotid artery

2. An extensor plantar reflex (extensor Babinski sign) occurs when there is damage to central nervous system motor pathways. The abnormal response is characterized by great toe extension (dorsiflexion) with the other toes fanning out.

3. Stocking glove sensory loss occurs in polyneuropathy related to:
   a. Diabetes mellitus
   b. Alcohol abuse
   c. Vitamin B_{12} deficiency

d. HIV infection
e. Syphilis

4. Proprioceptive loss occurs in neuropathy due to diabetes mellitus and vitamin B_{12} deficiency. Loss of proprioception is due to disease affecting the posterior spinal column or peripheral nerve or root.

E 178   **Answer: C**
C is correct because pemphigus is an autoimmune disease that causes formation of bullae (blisters).

■ **You Should Know**

1. Blistering diseases include pemphigus, bullous pemphigoid, dermatitis herpetiformis, erythema multiforme, porphyria cutanea tarda, and toxic epidermal necrolysis.

2. Nikolsky's sign is a mechanical sign that is often found in a patient with pemphigus. Application of pressure to the skin causes the superficial skin to separate from the deeper layers. The sign may be elicited on normal skin or at the margin of a blister.

3. Miliaria is a rash characterized by vesicles, papules, or pustules typically on the trunk and in intertriginous areas. It is most frequently noted in patients who live in hot, humid environments. It is due to plugging of eccrine sweat glands. Differential diagnosis includes drug rash and folliculitis.

E 179   **Answer: A**
A is correct because the diagnosis of candidiasis is made by potassium hydroxide (KOH) preparation on rash scrapings. Examination of the preparation shows budding yeasts with or without pseudohypha.

■ **You Should Know**

1. *Candida* are normal flora in the gastrointestinal and genitourinary tracts of humans.

2. Cutaneous candidiasis is particularly likely to occur in patients with diabetes mellitus or in obese persons who perspire freely.

3. Oral candidiasis (thrush) is seen in infants, those who wear dentures, patients on antibiotic therapy, chemotherapy, or radiation therapy to the head and neck, and in those patients with AIDS.

4. Esophageal candidiasis is an AIDS-defining illness. The patient may or may not have coexisting thrush.

5. Vulvovaginal candidiasis most often occurs in patients who have increased estrogen levels (e.g., pregnancy, oral contraceptive intake, or estrogen therapy). Other risk factors include diabetes mellitus, corticosteroid therapy, intrauterine devices, and diaphragm use.

6. Wood's lamp examination is used in the diagnosis of tinea capitis due to *Microsporum canis* or *Microsporum audouinii*, erythrasma, and porphyria cutanea tarda.

E 180   **Answer: A**
A is correct because complete right bundle branch block (RBBB) or incomplete right bundle branch block (RBBB) is present on electrocardiographic study in nearly all patients who have an atrial septal defect.

■ **You Should Know**

1. The electrocardiogram (ECG) in ventricular septal defect may be normal or may demonstrate left ventricular hypertrophy or biventricular hypertrophy depending upon the size of the shunt.

2. The electrocardiogram (ECG) in tetralogy typically demonstrates right ventricular hypertrophy and right axis deviation.

3. In the typical case of mitral valve prolapse the electrocardiogram (ECG) is normal.

4. Electrocardiogram (ECG) study in the patient with aortic valve stenosis commonly demonstrates left ventricular hypertrophy.

5. Complete right bundle branch block (RBBB) is, infrequently, considered to be a normal variant.

6. Pathologic causes of right bundle branch block (RBBB) include:
   a. Myocardial ischemia/infarction
   b. Myocarditis
   c. Cor pulmonale (conditions associated with chronically increased right ventricular pressure)
   d. Cardiomyopathy (e.g., sarcoid granulomas affecting the cardiac conduction system)
   e. Congenital heart disease (e.g., atrial septal defect)
   f. Degenerative disease of the conduction system in an otherwise healthy patient

7. Complete left bundle branch block (CLBBB) is rarely considered to be a normal variant.

8. Pathologic causes of complete left bundle branch block (CLBBB) include:
   a. Hypertension
   b. Myocardial ischemia/infarction
   c. Degenerative disease of the conduction system in an otherwise healthy patient
   d. Valvular disease
   e. Dilated cardiomyopathy

E 181   **Answer: D**
D is correct because intravenous adenosine is effective (90%) in terminating paroxysmal supraventricular tachycardia (PSVT). Further, it has a very short half-life (approximately 6 seconds). (The electrocardiogram in this patient demonstrates a regular, normal QRS tachycardia at a rate of 220/min.)

■ **You Should Know**

1. The initial treatment of paroxysmal supraventricular tachycardia (PSVT) is vagal stimulation including carotid sinus massage, Valsalva's maneuver, and splashing cold water on the face.

2. Never exert bilateral carotid sinus pressure at the same time.

3. Do not employ carotid sinus pressure if patient has a carotid artery bruit.

4. If paroxysmal supraventricular tachycardia (PSVT) is refractory to vagal stimulation, intravenous administration of adenosine is preferred. If the arrhythmia is refractory to adenosine, then the paroxysmal supraventricular tachycardia (PSVT) is often terminated by the intravenous administration of a calcium channel blocker (verapamil or diltiazem), beta-adrenergic blocker, or digoxin.

5. The primary mechanism of action of adenosine is to slow atrioventricular (AV) conduction. Therefore, transient atrioventricular (AV) block, even advanced block, may occur.

6. Adenosine may provoke bronchospasm in patients with reactive airways disease (i.e., asthma).

7. Tachycardias are generally categorized by normal QRS (<120 msec) or widened QRS (≥120 msec).

8. A narrow QRS suggests that the depolarization of the ventricles originates in or above the atrioventricular (AV) node.

9. A wide QRS suggests that the arrhythmia originates in the ventricle (i.e., ventricular tachycardia) *or* the arrhythmia is supraventricular with a pre-existing conduction defect or a rate-related aberrant conduction.

E 182   **Answer: E**
E is correct because tinea versicolor (TV) is a rash characterized by oval to round macules of various colors (white, orange-brown, and dark-brown) with overlying fine scales.

■ **You Should Know**

1. Tinea versicolor (TV) is a superficial infection caused by *Malassezia furfur*, a saprophytic yeast. Adolescents and young adults are most commonly affected.

2. Hot and humid weather, hyperhidrosis, skin oils, and immunosuppression appear to cause the clinical disease.

3. The diagnosis is confirmed by microscopic examination of skin scales using a 10% potassium hydroxide preparation.

4. Topical preparations (e.g., ketoconazole), may be used. Alternatively, oral medication (e.g., ketoconazole) may be used for therapy of extensive disease or resistant infection.

5. The rash of secondary syphilis is a symmetrical macular or popular eruption involving the entire trunk including palms and soles.

E 183   **Answer: D**
D is correct because approximately 75% of pregnant women have melasma, a hyperpigmentation that affects the cheeks, forehead, chin, and nose.

■ You Should Know

1. The cause of melasma is unknown.

2. Other factors that favor development of melasma include intake of oral contraceptives, exposure to the sun, and certain anti-epileptic medications.

3. Melasma associated with pregnancy usually recedes within 1 year after delivery.

4. In the differential diagnosis, other splotchy hyperpigmentation disorders, including acne, eczema, and contact dermatitis, are to be considered.

5. Therapy of melasma includes sunscreen, bleaching agents (hydroquinone, azelaic acid, tretinoin) and chemical peels.

E 184   **Answer: A**

A is correct because folliculitis due to *Pseudomonas aeruginosa* may occur from bathing in hot tubs that are inadequately chlorinated. Hot tub folliculitis usually resolves without treatment.

■ You Should Know

1. Folliculitis is a pustular eruption of the skin that is most commonly due to infection with *Staphylococcus aureus*.

2. Staphylococcal folliculitis is most commonly treated with topical agents including mupirocin or ethyl alcohol containing aluminum chloride.

3. Nasal carriage of *Staphylococcus* may cause recurrent folliculitis. Mupirocin ointment applied to the anterior nares is effective in eradicating *Staphylococcus aureus* colonization.

4. Less often, folliculitis is caused by infection by *Candida*, especially in patients taking broad-spectrum antibiotics.

5. Impetigo is a superficial vesiculopustular eruption that typically arises at sites of insect bites or abrasions. The pustules rupture causing a crusting with a golden appearance. *Staphylococcus aureus* and group A streptococci are the most common infecting organisms. Streptococcal impetigo may be associated with post-streptococcal glomerulonephritis in children.

E 185   **Answer: C**

C is correct because serologic tests are most commonly used for the diagnosis of coccidioidomycosis. These tests include tube precipitin antibodies (IgM) and complement-fixing antibodies.

■ You Should Know

1. Coccidioidomycosis is endemic in arid areas of the southwestern United States, Mexico, and Central and South Americas.

2. Coccidioidomycosis organisms grow a few inches under desert soil. Inhalation of conidia causes clinical infection.

3. The illness has a wide clinical spectrum, varying from insignificant illness to community-acquired pneumonia (CAP) to disseminated disease with meningitis, pulmonary cavitation, or abscess formation, and bone lesions.

4. Increased risk for disseminated disease occurs in the following:
   a. HIV-infected patients
   b. Diabetes mellitus patients
   c. Those on immunosuppressive or chemotherapy
   d. Pregnant women

5. Sputum culture is not routinely obtained for diagnosis. Dermal hypersensitivity to the coccidioidomycosis antigen remains for life. A positive skin test may reflect distant infection rather than current illness.

6. Healthy persons whose illness is limited to the chest do not need antifungal therapy. Antimicrobial therapy is for those who manifest progressive disease.

Part Two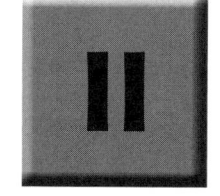

Performance: Gauging Your Test Success

The **PERFORMANCE** section provides you with clinical questions that relate to the medical topics in **ESSENTIALS.** In this carefully constructed manner, Performance is linked to Essentials and "You Should Know." As a result, you are learning much more about clinical medicine, not just learning isolated facts about a disease.

The questions are purposely not arranged by organ system. Rather, the questions are haphazard in their order in an effort to prepare the candidate for PANCE and PANRE questions. Thus, the test-book reader must quickly direct his or her critical thinking from Cardiology to Reproductive to Endocrinology, and so on.

Each question is labeled by Organ System. This text is constructed in a way so that you may retrieve questions related to a specific organ system. In order to promote the learning process, some questions have multiple organ system labels. For example, a question on endocarditis prophylaxis will be labeled "ID" (Infectious Disease) and "CV" (Cardiovascular). A question on melasma will be labeled DERM (Dermatology) and REPRO (Reproductive).

NOTE: There is only *ONE* best answer to a question in the Performance section.

Section One

Performance Test

CV

P 001 A 75-year-old man with chronic mitral regurgitation has dyspnea for 2 hours. Blood pressure is 90/70 mm Hg right arm sitting; respiratory rate, 28/min; and pulse of 130/min/irregularly irregular. Cardiac exam shows a dilated left ventricle and apical holosystolic murmur. Bibasilar rales are heard. Electrocardiography indicates atrial fibrillation. Chest radiograph shows bilateral pulmonary congestion. Which of the following is the preferred medicine to control the ventricular rate?

A. Digoxin
B. Verapamil
C. Metoprolol
D. Adenosine
E. Captopril

NEURO, PSY/LE

P 002 A 56-year-old man has dementia associated with chronic alcohol abuse. In addition to efforts to prevent continuing alcohol intake, which of the following therapeutic measures should be taken?

A. Oral administration of B-complex vitamins
B. Intravenous infusion of octreotide
C. Oral administration of levodopa
D. Oral administration of diazepam
E. Serial, subcutaneous injections of vitamin B_{12}

CV

P 003 A 14-year-old boy has a 2-week history of exertional dyspnea without associated cough, wheezing, or sputum production. Blood pressure is 120/80 mm Hg right arm sitting; pulse, 72/min/regular; and respirations, 17/min. A bisferiens carotid pulse is felt. An apical heave is felt. A diagnosis of hypertrophic cardiomyopathy is confirmed. In addition to administration of a diuretic, which of the following medications should be prescribed?

A. Oral digoxin
B. Oral verapamil
C. Oral captopril
D. Oral isosorbide dinitrate
E. Inhaled albuterol

NEURO

P 004 A 78-year-old man has a 2-month history of increasing memory loss and impaired judgment. He admits to recent urinary incontinence. Vital signs are normal. Exam shows an alert man with evidence of recent memory loss and impaired arithmetic calculations. Gait is wide based. Which of the following is the most likely diagnosis?

A. Alzheimer's disease
B. Chronic subdural hematoma
C. Normal pressure hydrocephalus
D. Encephalitis
E. Mad cow disease

HEME, GI/N

P 005 A 20-year old African American soldier is started on primaquine for malarial prophylaxis. One week later he notes asymptomatic jaundice. Laboratory values include a hemoglobin of 10 g/dL; total bilirubin, 3.8 mg/dL; and unconjugated bilirubin, 3.1 mg/dL. Which of the following is the most likely diagnosis?

A. *Mycoplasma* infection
B. Sickle cell anemia
C. Thalassemia
D. Glucose-6 phosphate dehydrogenase deficiency
E. Acute granulocytic leukemia

ENDO

P 006 A 56-year-old woman has a 2-month history of worsening memory, constipation, weakness, and cold intolerance. Exam shows a lethargic woman who is oriented to time and place. She has dry skin and thinning of the outer third of the eyelids. Deep tendon reflex relaxation is slow. Which of the following is an expected serum laboratory value?

A. Fasting blood sugar 42 mg/dL
B. Sodium 118 mEq/L
C. Total cholesterol 146 mg/dL
D. Thyroid-stimulating hormone 22 microU/mL
E. Albumin 2.0 g/dL

CV

P 007 A 54-year-old man with chronic hypertension has a 2-week history of exertional breathlessness without associated cough, wheezing, or sputum production. There is no history of allergy. Blood pressure is 150/90 mm Hg sitting; pulse, 90/min/regular; and respiratory rate, 20/min. Exam shows an apical lift and S4 gallop, but no murmur is present. Bibasilar crackles are heard. Which of the following is the most likely diagnosis?

A. Asthma
B. Psychogenic dyspnea
C. Diastolic heart failure
D. Cystic fibrosis
E. Dissection of the aorta

CV

P 008   A 57-year-old man has a 3-week history of increasing exertional dyspnea without cough, wheezing, or chest discomfort. At rest, vital signs and cardiopulmonary examination are normal. During treadmill exercise testing, the patient has dyspnea without anginal discomfort. At that time, the electrocardiogram shows horizontal ST segment depression. Which of the following is the most likely diagnosis?

A. Unstable angina pectoris
B. Variant angina pectoris
C. Anginal equivalent
D. Noncardiac dyspnea
E. Anxiety reaction

CV

P 009   A 14-year-old boy has anterior chest pressure radiating down the left arm and shortness of breath when he is playing basketball. The symptoms cease within 3 minutes of rest. Blood pressure is 130/90 mm Hg sitting; pulse, 70/min/regular; and respirations, 18/min. Examination shows an apical heave, 2/6 left lower sternal border ejection murmur, and apical S4 gallop. There is no chest wall tenderness. Which of the following is the most likely diagnosis?

A. Anomalous origin of a coronary artery
B. Atherosclerotic heart disease
C. Mitral valve prolapse
D. Hypertrophic obstructive cardiomyopathy
E. Rheumatic mitral regurgitation

ENDO, MS

P 010   A 43 year old man with a history of gout is to start therapy for dyslipidemia. Which of the following medications should not be prescribed?

A. Niacin
B. Cholestyramine
C. Simvastatin
D. Clofibrate
E. Ezetimibe

CV

P 011   Five minutes after inhaling cocaine, an 18-year-old man has severe anterior chest pressure and sweating for which he is taken to the emergency department. The patient is alert, pink, and tremulous. Blood pressure is 230/120 mm Hg recumbent; pulse rate, 130/min/regular; and respiratory rate, 28/min. Lung examination is normal. An apical S4 gallop is heard. Electrocardiography shows ST segment elevation in leads V1-V4. In addition to nitrates, which of the following medications should be given?

A. Propranolol
B. Verapamil
C. Hydralazine
D. Adenosine
E. Captopril

GI/N

P 012 A 57-year-old man with a long history of alcohol abuse has cirrhosis. He suddenly vomits very large amounts of red blood. Which of the following is the preferred initial therapeutic measure?

A. Insertion of Sengstaken-Blakemore tube
B. Intravenous administration of metoprolol
C. Intravenous administration of octreotide
D. Rectal administration of lactulose
E. Nasogastric administration of omeprazole

CV

P 013 A 78-year-old man has stable angina pectoris and chronic hypertension for which he takes lisinopril, verapamil, and nitroglycerin. The patient suddenly has a syncopal episode lasting 30 seconds. Blood pressure is 90/70 mm Hg; pulse, 46/min; and respiratory rate, 24/min. Electrocardiogram reveals Mobitz I atrioventricular block. Which of the following is the most likely cause of the syncope?

A. Adverse effect of verapamil
B. Vasovagal reaction
C. Orthostatic hypotension
D. Hypovolemia
E. Carotid artery stenosis

HEME, CV

P 014 A 66-year-old man has a 2-week history of increasing facial swelling. Vital signs are normal. The face is suffused and edematous. There is dilatation of arm and chest veins. The central venous pressure is elevated. There is no peripheral edema. Bilateral cervical, axillary, and inguinal nodes are felt. Which of the following is the most likely diagnosis?

A. Sarcoidosis
B. Non-Hodgkin's lymphoma
C. Right heart failure
D. Constrictive pericarditis
E. Angioneurotic edema

CV, GI/N

P 015 A 47-year-old woman has a 2-week history of increasing abdominal distention and peripheral edema. Four years earlier she had received chest radiotherapy for carcinoma of the breast. Blood pressure is 100/70 mm Hg sitting; pulse, 96/min/regular; and respiratory rate, 18/min. Central venous pressure is elevated. Lungs are clear. No murmur or gallop is heard. Ascites and bilateral ankle edema are present. Which of the following is the most likely diagnosis?

A. Right heart failure
B. Pulmonary embolism
C. Mitral valve stenosis
D. Constrictive pericarditis
E. Superior vena cava syndrome

CV

P 016 A 68-year-old woman with chronic hypertension suddenly has severe, tearing pain in the anterior chest lasting 30 minutes. Supine blood pressure is 180/100 mm Hg left arm and 140/90 mm Hg right arm. Pulse is 100/min/regular and respiratory rate is 30/min. A new 2/6 right sternal border diastolic decrescendo murmur is heard. Which of the following is the test most likely to establish the diagnosis?

A. Transesophageal echocardiogram
B. Aortogram
C. Chest radiograph
D. Cardiac enzyme profile
E. Ventilation perfusion scan

GI/N

P 017 A 35-year-old man has long-standing Crohn's disease. He now has 3 hours of right upper quadrant abdominal pain associated with nausea without vomiting. Blood pressure is 120/82 mm Hg recumbent; pulse, 100/min/regular; and respiratory rate 18/min. Examination shows the patient to be nonicteric. The abdomen is flat and symmetrical. Moderate epigastric tenderness is present. No mass is felt and bowel sounds are hypoactive. Serum laboratory values: amylase, 200 units/L; alanine aminotransferase, 106 units/L; alkaline phosphatase, 130 units/L. Which of the following is the most likely diagnosis?

A. Acute cholecystitis
B. Acute pancreatitis
C. Peritonitis secondary to bowel perforation
D. Mesenteric ischemia
E. Acute intermittent porphyria

GI/N, DERM

P 018 A 45-year-old woman has a 1-month history of fatigue and a 2-week history of pruritus without rash. She takes no medication. Vital signs are normal. Examination shows xanthomas around the eyelids and slight hepatomegaly. Serum alkaline phosphatase is 300 units/L, gamma-glutamyl transpeptidase is 130 units/L, and total bilirubin is 1.2 mg/dL. Which of the following is the most likely diagnosis?

A. Metastatic carcinoma to bone
B. Primary biliary cirrhosis
C. Carcinoma of the pancreas
D. Chronic fatigue syndrome
E. Ischemic hepatic insufficiency

ENDO, GU

P 019 A 45-year-old man with type 1 diabetes mellitus now has proteinuria. Serum creatinine is 1.0 mg/dL and blood urea nitrogen is 18 mg/dL. Blood pressure is 140/80 mm Hg sitting. Which of the following is recommended therapy?

    A. Initiate thiazide therapy
    B. Initiate angiotensin-converting enzyme inhibitor therapy
    C. Observation for onset of azotemia
    D. Initiate hydralazine therapy
    E. Reduce insulin dosage

CV, ID

P 020 A 40-year-old woman has the acute onset of severe, anterior chest pain that is eased by sitting forward and increased during swallowing and changes in body position. For the past 3 weeks, the patient has had fatigue and generalized arthralgia. Examination shows the presence of a pericardial friction rub. White blood cell count is 2200/microL. Which of the following is the most likely diagnosis?

    A. Pericarditis due to Coxsackie virus
    B. Pericarditis due to *Staphylococcus* infection
    C. Systemic lupus erythematosus
    D. Constrictive pericarditis
    E. Superior vena cava syndrome

NEURO, ENDO, CV

P 021 A 65-year-old man has lightheadedness when arising from bed. In the sitting position blood pressure is 130/70 with pulse of 70/min/regular. Standing blood pressure is 100/50 mm Hg and pulse is 71/min/regular. Oral temperature is 98.6°F. Which of the following is the most likely etiology of the patient's symptoms?

    A. Hypovolemia due to excessive diuresis
    B. Addison's disease
    C. Autonomic insufficiency
    D. Pheochromocytoma
    E. Gram-negative sepsis

MS

P 022 A 57-year-old woman is to begin alendronate as treatment for osteoporosis. Which of the following instructions should be given to the patient?

    A. Take medication at bedtime
    B. Do not eat for 60 minutes after taking medication
    C. Take medication with an aluminum-containing antacid
    D. Stand or sit upright for 30 minutes after taking medication
    E. Check daily for signs of purpura

ENDO

P 023　Niacin therapy is initiated for dyslipidemia in a 56-year-old man with type I diabetes mellitus. Which of the following instructions should be given to the patient?

　　A. Insulin dosage may increase due to hyperglycemic effect of niacin
　　B. Proteinuria may occur as a side effect of medication
　　C. Do not ingest niacin within 2 hours of insulin administration
　　D. Take niacin with psyllium preparation
　　E. Angioedema is a common adverse effect of medication

NEURO

P 024　A 48-year-old woman has a 2-month history of progressively worsening tremor of both hands. Examination shows a marked tremor when holding a glass of water with a stationary outstretched arm. The tremor worsens when bringing the glass to her lips. Neurologic examination is otherwise normal. Which of the following is the preferred initial therapy?

　　A. Levodopa
　　B. Prostigmine
　　C. Diazepam
　　D. Propranolol
　　E. Carbamazepine

CV

P 025　A 57-year-old man has a history of remote myocardial infarction. He has an elevated serum C-reactive protein level that places him in the upper quartile compared to normal values. The patient should be advised that he is at increased risk for which of the following?

　　A. Carcinoma of the colon
　　B. Venous thrombosis
　　C. Rheumatoid arthritis
　　D. Recurrent myocardial infarction
　　E. Glaucoma

GI/N, DERM

P 026　A 44-year-old woman has fatigue and generalized pruritus. A diagnosis of primary biliary cirrhosis is made. Presence in the serum of antibodies to which of the following is most likely?

　　A. Smooth muscle
　　B. Mitochondria
　　C. Acetylcholine receptors
　　D. Gastric parietal cells
　　E. Endotoxin

GI/N

P 027 A 56-year-old man has cirrhosis due to chronic alcohol abuse. An increase in which of the following serum levels raises suspicion of hepatocellular carcinoma?

A. Beta carotene
B. Alpha-fetoprotein
C. Alpha-tocopherol
D. Beta globin
E. CA 125

CV, HEME

P 028 A 36-year-old woman has acute pericarditis. A diagnosis of systemic lupus erythematosus is made. Which of the following laboratory values would be expected in this patient?

A. Platelet count 625,000/microL
B. Hemoglobin 17 g/dL
C. White blood cell count 2100/microL
D. Fasting blood sugar 170 mg/dL
E. Serum ferritin 120 ng/mL

ENDO, CV

P 029 A 40-year-old woman has a 1-month history of paroxysmal sweating and palpitations. Examination shows a sitting blood pressure 180/120 mm Hg and pulse 100/min/regular. In the standing position, blood pressure is 150/104 mm Hg with pulse of 114/min. Which of the following is the most likely etiology of the hypertension?

A. Essential hypertension
B. Hypercortisolism
C. Primary hyperaldosteronism
D. Pheochromocytoma
E. Coarctation of the aorta

ENDO, GI/N

P 030 A 60-year-old woman has a 2-month history of fatigue, nausea, anorexia, and a 6-pound weight loss. Which of the following is the preferred laboratory test to establish a diagnosis of Addison's disease?

A. Dexamethasone suppression test
B. Plasma renin activity
C. Schilling test
D. Cosyntropin stimulation test
E. 24-hour urinary sodium excretion value

NEURO, CV

P 031 A 79-year-old woman faints while sitting in a chair. Upon awakening she has mild nausea. Examination in the emergency department shows the patient to be alert and pink. Blood pressure is 110/70 mm Hg right arm recumbent, pulse is 96/min/regular, and respiratory rate is 17/min. Which of the following is the preferred initial diagnostic test?

A. Electroencephalogram
B. Ambulatory cardiac monitoring
C. CT imaging of the brain
D. Carotid ultrasound study
E. Serum creatine kinase and troponin levels

PUL, CV

P 032 A 54-year-old man with a 40 pack-year history of cigarette smoking has a chronic productive cough and dyspnea. In the past 2 weeks, he has swelling of both lower legs and abdominal distention. Examination shows elevated central venous pressure, an enlarged, smooth tender liver, and 2+ bilateral lower leg edema. Which of the following is the most likely diagnosis?

A. Left heart failure
B. Constrictive pericarditis
C. Right heart failure
D. Superior vena cava syndrome
E. High cardiac output heart failure

PSY/LE, ENDO

P 033 Lithium therapy is initiated in a 27-year-old woman who has bipolar disorder. Which of the following should be followed in the management of the patient?

A. Obtain serum electrolyte values every 3 to 4 months
B. Obtain thyroid function values every 3 to 4 months
C. Advise patient to take oral potassium supplement
D. Obtain lipid profile values every 3 to 4 months
E. Advise patient to take medication on an empty stomach

NEURO

P 034 A 76-year-old woman has had three episodes of blurred vision in her right eye in the past week. Each episode lasts approximately 2 minutes and is described as "a curtain coming down over my eye." There are no associated symptoms. Vital signs are normal. When the patient is asymptomatic, the neurologic examination is normal. Which of the following is the most likely diagnosis?

A. Multiple sclerosis
B. Vertebrobasilar artery insufficiency
C. Amaurosis fugax
D. Petit mal seizures
E. Transient 3rd degree atrioventricular block

PSY/LE

P 035 A 6-year-old boy has impulsivity, distractiveness, and inattentiveness that cause behavioral problems in school. He now has involuntary, repetitive momentary coughs and facial grimacing and is beginning to repeat sentences made by the teacher. Which of the following is the most likely diagnosis?

A. Oppositional defiant behavior syndrome
B. Tourette's syndrome
C. Fetal alcohol syndrome
D. Fragile X syndrome
E. Hyperactive autism

DERM, GI/N

P 036 A 2-year-old girl has a 3-week history of recurrent hives, flushing, and diarrhea approximately 30 minutes after eating. The mother is instructed to keep a diary of the child's food intake. Which of the following is least likely to precipitate the symptoms?

A. Wheat
B. Eggs
C. Soy
D. Milk
E. Oats

CV, NEURO

P 037 Immediately after witnessing a serious automobile accident, a 17-year-old woman has a cold sweat and nausea followed by fainting. Pulse is 32/min/regular and blood pressure is 70/40 mm Hg recumbent. Which of the following is the pathophysiologic mechanism causing the faint?

A. Orthostatic hypotension
B. Heightened vagal tone
C. Increased ventricular preload
D. Systemic hypoxemia
E. Increased prostaglandin secretion

PUL, CV

P 038 A 61-year-old woman with a 40 pack-year history of cigarette smoking has chronic dyspnea and productive cough. In the past 3 weeks she has worsening breathlessness, swelling of both lower legs, and abdominal distention. Examination shows central cyanosis, elevated central venous pressure, an enlarged, tender, smooth liver, and 2+ bilateral ankle edema. Which of the following is the primary pathophysiologic abnormality?

A. Decreased right ventricular preload
B. Increased cardiac output
C. Respiratory alkalosis
D. Pulmonary hypertension
E. Increased mean left atrial pressure

GI/N

P 039 A newborn infant fails to pass meconium followed by progressive abdominal distention and vomiting. Which of the following is the definitive diagnostic test?

A. Abdominal ultrasonography
B. Inferior mesenteric arteriography
C. Spiral CT scan of the abdomen
D. Anorectal manometry
E. Small bowel contrast study via nasogastric tube

EENT, MS

P 040 A 34-year-old woman has been taking prednisone for 3 years as therapy for rheumatoid arthritis. She now notes the slow onset of painless, bilateral persistently blurred vision in both eyes. Which of the following is the most likely cause of the ocular symptoms?

A. Vertebrobasilar artery insufficiency
B. Open-angle glaucoma
C. Uveitis
D. Cataracts
E. Myasthenia gravis

PSY/LE, REPRO

P 041 A 21-year-old woman is started on lithium therapy for the treatment of bipolar disorder. Which of the following instructions should be given to the patient?

A. Ingest a high-carbohydrate, low-fat diet
B. Avoid pregnancy while taking lithium
C. Avoid nonsteroidal anti-inflammatory medicines
D. Advise patient of risk of nasal polyps
E. Advise patient to take daily oral potassium supplement

GI/N, DERM

P 042 A 67-year-old woman has a 1-month history of 12-pound weight loss, anorexia, progressive weakness, and new skin lesions. Examination shows a wasted woman with bilateral axillary patches of thickened dark brown skin having prominent skin lines. Which of the following is the most likely diagnosis?

A. Adenocarcinoma of the stomach
B. Addison's disease
C. Diabetes insipidus
D. Adenocarcinoma of the ovary
E. Adenocarcinoma of the pancreas

GI/N, GU

P 043 A 6-year-old child has cholera with severe diarrhea. Which of the following laboratory abnormalities is the most likely to occur?

A. Hyperglycemia
B. Hypokalemia
C. Hypernatremia
D. Metabolic alkalosis
E. Hypertriglyceridemia

ID

P 044 A 16-year-old girl has a 3-day history of sore throat, fever, and malaise. Examination shows tonsillar inflammation with white exudates and diffuse adenopathy. A diagnosis of infectious mononucleosis is made. Which of the following is the most likely complication?

A. Aseptic meningitis
B. Endocarditis
C. Nephrotic syndrome
D. Megaloblastic anemia
E. Uveitis

EENT

P 045 An 18-year-old woman is prescribed contact lens in place of eyeglasses. She should be advised that the most frequent complication is which of the following?

A. Optic neuritis
B. Adenovirus conjunctivitis
C. Corneal ulceration
D. Herpes simplex keratitis
E. Closed-angle glaucoma

MS, GI/N

P 046 A 40-year-old woman has a 2-year history of Raynaud's phenomenon. She now has heartburn and dysphagia to both solids and liquids. Vital signs are normal. Examination shows thickening of the skin of the fingers with loss of creases. Which of the following is the most likely diagnosis?

A. Sjögren's syndrome
B. Achalasia
C. Squamous cell carcinoma of the esophagus
D. Carcinoma of the lung with paraneoplastic syndrome
E. Scleroderma

ID, NEURO

P 047 An 18-year-old man living in Connecticut has the sudden onset of bilateral Bell's palsy. Two months earlier he had a flulike illness with fever, chills, and myalgia. At that time, he had noted a slightly raised, red rash on his thigh. Which of the following tests is the preferred initial diagnostic test?

A. ELISA test
B. Biopsy of skin in area of rash, with culture
C. Assay of serum immunoglobulin A
D. Dark field microscopic examination of blood
E. Blood culture in anaerobic medium

HEME

P 048 A 55-year-old man with aggressive stage IV non-Hodgkin's lymphoma is to begin chemotherapy. Initiation of which of the following prophylactic interventions is indicated?

A. Oral acetazolamide
B. Oral ammonium chloride
C. Oral allopurinol
D. Intravenous hypotonic glucose
E. Intravenous lidocaine

PUL, GI/N

P 049 A 43-year-old African American woman has a 2-week history of malaise and dry cough. Examination shows bilateral enlargement of the parotid glands and enlargement of the submandibular and axillary lymph nodes. Chest radiograph shows bilateral hilar enlargement. Which of the following is an expected serum abnormality?

A. Elevated immunoglobulin A
B. Elevated angiotensin-converting enzyme
C. Reduced calcium
D. Elevated gastrin
E. Reduced norepinephrine

EENT

P 050 An 18-year-old woman is to start wearing contact lens for correction of a refractive error. Which of the following is the proper advice to be given to the patient?

A. Hard lens are better tolerated than soft lens
B. Sterilization is best accomplished through antibiotic solutions
C. Avoid extended wear of the soft lens
D. At 3-month intervals, do not wear contact lens for 2 weeks
E. Disposable lens do not cause corneal ulceration

ENDO, EENT, NEURO

P 051 A 66-year-old man awakens and suddenly is aware of double vision when both eyes are open. Vital signs are normal. Examination shows an alert, cooperative man. There is ptosis of the left eyelid with lateral deviation of the eye. The pupil size of the affected eye is normal. Which of the following is the most likely underlying disorder?

   A. Cerebral aneurysm
   B. Diabetes mellitus
   C. Wernicke's encephalopathy
   D. Cataract
   E. Hypothyroidism

CV

P 052 A 78-year-old man with chronic hypertension has the acute onset of severe, tearing upper posterior chest pain lasting 40 minutes. Blood pressure is 170/100 mm Hg right arm recumbent and 130/80 mm Hg left arm recumbent. Pulse is 110/min/regular and respiratory rate 30/min. Electrocardiography shows left ventricular hypertrophy. Which of the following is the most likely diagnosis?

   A. Acute myocardial infarction
   B. Acute occlusion of the innominate artery
   C. Superior vena cava syndrome
   D. Acute dissection of the thoracic aorta
   E. Subclavian steal syndrome

NEURO, EENT

P 053 A 71-year-old woman has had three episodes of blurred vision in her left eye in the past week. Each episode lasts 1 to 2 minutes followed by spontaneous return of normal vision. There are no associated symptoms. Vital signs are normal. Neurologic examination is normal. Which of the following is the preferred initial intervention?

   A. Initiate propranolol therapy
   B. Obtain serum anti-phospholipid antibody level
   C. Perform duplex carotid artery ultrasound
   D. Obtain erythrocyte sedimentation rate value
   E. Trial of sumatriptan when episode recurs

MS

P 054 A 37-year-old woman has been taking prednisone for 4 years as therapy for rheumatoid arthritis. Bone density study now shows significant osteopenia. In addition to oral calcium supplementation, which of the following is recommended?

   A. Initiate therapy with a thiazide diuretic
   B. Initiate therapy with fluoride
   C. Initiate therapy with a bisphosphonate
   D. Obtain 24-hour urinary calcium level
   E. Initiate high-protein diet

CV, GU

P 055 A 78-year-old man has chronic systolic heart failure for which he takes digoxin, furosemide, and lisinopril. His electrocardiogram now shows frequent ventricular ectopic beats due to digoxin toxicity. Which of the following is the most likely precipitating factor causing the toxicity?

A. Metabolic acidosis
B. Hypokalemia
C. Hypermagnesemia
D. Hyponatremia
E. Hyperosmolality

GU, CV

P 056 A 66-year-old man has a 3-hour history of increasing weakness. He takes lisinopril for hypertension and, for the past 2 days, has used artificial salt on his food. In the emergency department, serum potassium is 6.8 mEq/L. The serum creatinine is 1.3 mg/dL and blood urea nitrogen is 22 mg/dL. The electrocardiogram shows peaked T waves. Which of the following is the preferred initial therapy?

A. Emergent hemodialysis
B. Administration of intravenous calcium
C. Administration of intravenous glucose and insulin
D. Sodium polystyrene sulfonate enema
E. Administration of intravenous epinephrine

GI/N, DERM

P 057 A 52-year-old man has a 4-month history of progressive exertional breathlessness without associated cough or angina pectoris. He now has dysphagia to both solids and liquids. Blood pressure is 140/90 mm Hg sitting; pulse, 96/min/regular; and respiratory rate, 28/min. Examination shows thickening of the skin of the face and hands. Telangiectasia are noted on the face. Chest radiograph shows diffuse pulmonary fibrosis. Which of the following is the most likely diagnosis?

A. Sarcoidosis
B. Chronic pulmonary embolic disease
C. Asbestosis
D. Scleroderma
E. Silo-Piller's disease

PUL

P 058 A 42-year-old man has exertional dyspnea and dry cough due to sarcoidosis. Chest radiograph shows diffuse interstitial fibrosis. Which of the following systemic arterial blood values would be expected?

A. pH 7.48, PaO_2 66 mm Hg, $PaCO_2$ 28 mm Hg
B. pH 7.40, PaO_2 100 mm Hg, $PaCO_2$ 40 mm Hg
C. pH 7.48, PaO_2 100 mm Hg, $PaCO_2$ 48 mm Hg
D. pH 7.34, PaO_2 66 mm Hg, $PaCO_2$ 28 mm Hg
E. pH 7.34, PaO_2 100 mm Hg, $PaCO_2$ 28 mm Hg

PUL

P 059 A 66-year-old man has exertional dyspnea and dry cough due to idiopathic diffuse pulmonary fibrosis. Which of the following is an expected abnormality on pulmonary function testing?

A. Decreased forced expiratory volume 1 sec/forced vital capacity ratio (FEV 1 sec/FVC)
B. Increased residual volume
C. Decreased carbon monoxide diffusing capacity
D. Decreased forced expiratory flow rate
E. Increased vital capacity

HEME

P 060 Presence of which of the following would be expected on examination of a peripheral blood smear in a patient who has pernicious anemia?

A. Microcytosis
B. Hypersegmented neutrophiles
C. Target red blood cells
D. Blast cells
E. Increased number of platelets

HEME, MS, GI/N

P 061 After having had diffuse joint aching for 4 days, a 6-year-old girl now has diffuse abdominal pain and a rash on her legs. Vital signs are normal. Abdominal examination shows diffuse tenderness with normal bowel sounds. Palpable purpura is noted on both legs. Urinalysis shows 10 to 15 RBCs per high-power field and red blood cell casts. Which of the following is the most likely diagnosis?

A. Systemic lupus erythematosus
B. Serum sickness
C. Acute rheumatic fever
D. Endocarditis
E. Henoch-Schönlein purpura

NEURO, HEME

P 062 A 73-year-old woman has paresthesia and ataxia. Peripheral blood examination shows macrocytosis. The serum vitamin B_{12} level is borderline abnormal. Which of the following serum values should be obtained in order to confirm a diagnosis of pernicious anemia?

A. C-reactive protein
B. 5 Hydroxytryptamine
C. Methylmalonic acid
D. Gastrin
E. Anti-phospholipid antibody

CV

P 063 A 31-year-old woman with Marfan's syndrome has the sudden onset of severe, ripping anterior chest pain followed by collapse. Blood pressure is 70/40 mm Hg both arms recumbent; pulse, 140/min/regular; and respiratory rate, 38/min. The patient is cold and pale. Central venous pressure is elevated. Which of the following is the preferred initial diagnostic test?

A. Aortography
B. Positron emission tomography
C. Transesophageal echocardiography
D. Thoracentesis
E. Magnetic resonance venography

PUL, ID

P 064 A 66-year-old man has an acute exacerbation of chronic bronchitis for which tetracycline is prescribed. Which of the following is proper counseling to be given to the patient?

A. Take medication with milk
B. Do not take medication with antacids
C. Medication may cause ecchymosis
D. Medication may cause rectal bleeding
E. Avoid intake of tea while taking medication

CV

P 065 A 69-year-old woman has the sudden onset of tearing anterior chest pain lasting 1 hour. Blood pressure is 180/110 mm Hg both arms recumbent; pulse, 120/min/regular; and respiratory rate, 24/min. Central venous pressure is normal. Cardiac examination shows an apical lift and new 2/6 left sternal border diastolic murmur. In addition to intravenous nitroprusside, which of the following medicines should be administered intravenously?

A. Hydralazine
B. Metoprolol
C. Diazoxide
D. Low molecular weight heparin
E. Tirofiban

HEME, NEURO

P 066 Presence of which of the following differentiates pernicious anemia from folic acid deficiency anemia?

A. Hypersegmented neutrophiles
B. Abnormal position sense
C. Megaloblastic bone marrow
D. Hypertension
E. Anti-phospholipid antibodies

GI/N

P 067 Which of the following is proper counseling for a patient who has Crohn's disease with extensive involvement of the small bowel?

A. Avoid acetaminophen intake
B. Avoid cephalosporin intake
C. Receive monthly vitamin B_{12} injections
D. Receive annual pneumococcal vaccine
E. Avoid the sun's direct rays as much as possible

GI/N, HEME

P 068 Which of the following is the mechanism by which gastrectomy causes megaloblastic anemia?

A. Dumping syndrome
B. Alkalinity in the small bowel
C. Lack of intrinsic factor production
D. Reduced parasympathomimetic intestinal tone
E. Lack of gastrin production

GI/N, PUL, ENDO

P 069 Which of the following conditions is associated with hypertrophic osteoarthropathy?

A. Hyperthyroidism
B. Crohn's disease
C. Angiodysplasia of the colon
D. Acromegaly
E. Hyperparathyroidism

CV

P 070 Which of the following is the pathophysiologic basis for the increased pulse pressure associated with aging?

A. Decreased arterial compliance
B. Increased stroke volume
C. Decreased ventricular contractility
D. Decreased preload
E. Decreased cardiac output

CV

P 071 A 76-year-old asymptomatic man has had four blood pressure measurements over a 2-week period. The blood pressure range is 158–170/70–78 mm Hg. He takes no medication. Which of the following is the preferred management?

A. Initiate angiotensin-converting enzyme inhibitor therapy
B. No medicinal therapy
C. Initiate thiazide therapy
D. Initiate fish oil supplementation
E. Initiate beta-adrenergic blocker therapy

HEME, NEURO

P 072 A 77-year-old woman has a 2-month history of bilateral leg paresthesias. Blood examination shows anemia, macrocytosis, and hypersegmented neutrophiles. Which of the following neurologic signs would be expected to be abnormal in this patient?

   A. Pupillary response to light
   B. Extraocular muscle movement
   C. Romberg test
   D. Stereognosis
   E. Cranial nerve VII function

ENDO, CV

P 073 A 79-year-old woman has a 1-month history of generalized weakness and a 6-pound weight loss. She now presents in the emergency department with new onset atrial fibrillation. Which of the following is the most likely diagnosis?

   A. Adrenal insufficiency
   B. Hypercortisolism
   C. Hyperthyroidism
   D. Hyperparathyroidism
   E. Zollinger-Ellison syndrome

NEURO, ENDO, CV

P 074 A 67-year-old man with type 1 diabetes mellitus has symptomatic orthostatic hypotension. His medications include insulin, aspirin, and simvastatin. Which of the following is the most likely pathophysiologic mechanism causing the orthostatic hypotension?

   A. Hypovolemia
   B. Autonomic insufficiency
   C. Decreased number of serotonin receptors
   D. Decreased cardiac output
   E. Metabolic acidosis

NEURO, CV

P 075 A 54-year-old woman has lightheadedness and graying of vision upon arising from bed. Blood pressure is 114/72 mm Hg with pulse 78/min in the sitting position. Upon arising, blood pressure is 92/58 with pulse 106/min. Which of the following is the most likely cause?

   A. Autonomic insufficiency
   B. Decreased left ventricular compliance
   C. Decreased serum norepinephrine level
   D. Hypovolemia
   E. Hypo-osmolar serum

NEURO, ENDO, CV

P 076 A 49-year-old man faints when arising from bed. Blood pressure is 118/74 mm Hg with pulse 84/min in the sitting position. Upon arising blood pressure is 78/48 mm Hg with pulse of 85/min. Which of the following is the most likely underlying diagnosis?

  A. Chronic adrenal insufficiency
  B. Excessive diuresis
  C. Diabetes mellitus
  D. Nonfunctioning pituitary adenoma
  E. Bleeding gastric ulcer

CV

P 077 Which of the following is the pathophysiologic mechanism that causes an increased plasma Nt-BNP level in patients who have heart failure?

  A. Decreased glomerular filtration rate
  B. Decreased systemic vascular resistance
  C. Ventricular wall stretching
  D. Stimulation of baroreceptors
  E. Decreased plasma renin activity

PUL, CV

P 078 A 65-year- old man who has a long history of cigarette smoking and a 7-year history of hypertension now has worsening dyspnea over 1 week. Which of the following is the best indicator to exclude heart failure?

  A. Normal central venous pressure
  B. Absence of gallop sound
  C. Normal urine osmolality
  D. Normal plasma Nt-BNP
  E. Normal serum C-reactive protein

ENDO, PUL

P 079 Which of the following is the most likely source of ectopic adrenocorticotrophic hormone (ACTH)?

  A. Villous adenoma of the colon
  B. Medullary carcinoma of the thyroid
  C. Parathyroid adenoma
  D. Gastrinoma
  E. Small cell carcinoma of lung

PUL, ID

P 080 A 32-year-old man with cystic fibrosis has an acute, extensive pneumonia. Which of the following is the most likely infecting organism?

  A. *Escherichia coli*
  B. Fusiform bacilli
  C. Respiratory syncytial virus
  D. *Chlamydia trachomatis*
  E. *Pseudomonas aeruginosa*

CV, HEME

P 081 Heparin therapy is initiated in a 67-year-old woman for treatment of deep venous thrombosis. Which of the following should be performed after 5 days of anticoagulation?

- A. Prothrombin time
- B. Platelet count
- C. White blood cell count
- D. Serum sodium level
- E. Arterial blood gas determination

PUL

P 082 Which of the following is a pulmonary complication of cystic fibrosis?

- A. Diffuse interstitial fibrosis
- B. Granulomatous infiltration
- C. Eisenmenger syndrome
- D. Bronchiectasis
- E. Bullae formation

PSY/LE, CV

P 083 Lithium therapy is initiated in a 36-year-old man for treatment of bipolar disorder. He should be counseled that which of the following medicines will increase lithium blood levels?

- A. Aspirin
- B. Acetaminophen
- C. Meclizine
- D. Verapamil
- E. Hydrochlorothiazide

PSY/LE, REPRO

P 084 Lithium therapy is to be initiated in a 32-year-old woman for treatment of bipolar disorder. Which of the following is proper counseling for the patient?

- A. Reduce ingestion of potassium-containing foods
- B. Avoid pregnancy
- C. Check complete blood count every 4 months
- D. Wear gloves when holding frozen foods
- E. Check blood pressure every 2 months

NEURO, EENT

P 085 Presence of which of the following differentiates the visual symptoms of unilateral carotid artery stenosis from migraine?

- A. Unilateral character of visual symptoms
- B. Symptoms last more than 2 hours
- C. Presence of "stars" and "sparks" in visual fields
- D. Association with photophobia
- E. Association with nausea and vomiting

EENT, ENDO

P 086　Intake of which of the following medicines is most likely to be associated with premature cataract formation?

　　A. Prednisone
　　B. Lithium
　　C. Diazepam
　　D. Radioactive iodine
　　E. Estrogen/progesterone combination

DERM, GI/N

P 087　A 56-year-old woman develops acanthosis nigricans in the axillary areas. Which of the following is the most likely associated condition?

　　A. Chronic adrenal insufficiency
　　B. Hyperthyroidism
　　C. Crohn's disease
　　D. Acromegaly
　　E. Gastric adenocarcinoma

DERM, ENDO

P 088　Which of the following is a pathophysiologic abnormality associated with acanthosis nigricans?

　　A. Deficiency of bile salts
　　B. Tissue insulin resistance
　　C. Ectopic adrenocorticotrophic hormone production
　　D. Defective glycogenolysis
　　E. Increased somatostatin secretion

DERM, ID

P 089　Which of the following is the typical skin rash associated with Lyme disease?

　　A. Erythema multiforme
　　B. Erythema migrans
　　C. Erysipelas
　　D. Dermatitis herpetiformis
　　E. Erythema marginatum

HEME, GU

P 090　A 14-year-old girl has acute leukemia for which chemotherapy is to be initiated. Which of the following is the appropriate prophylactic medication to be given to the patient in order to prevent tumor lysis syndrome?

　　A. Oral theophylline
　　B. Inhaled albuterol
　　C. Intravenous potassium
　　D. Oral allopurinol
　　E. Intramuscular glucagons

PUL

P 091 Presence of which of the following differentiates idiopathic pulmonary fibrosis from chronic bronchitis?

A. Decreased systemic arterial PaO_2
B. Respiratory acidosis
C. Increased tidal volume
D. Normal FEV 1 sec/FVC ratio
E. Normal carbon monoxide diffusing capacity

HEME, GU

P 092 A 22-year-old man with bulky non-Hodgkin's lymphoma is to start chemotherapy. Prevention of which of the following is the reason to give prophylactic allopurinol to the patient?

A. Dilated cardiomyopathy
B. Hyperuricemic nephropathy
C. Seizures
D. Increased anion gap metabolic acidosis
E. Mesenteric ischemia

CV

P 093 A 77-year-old man is diagnosed with chronic systolic heart failure. He is in normal sinus rhythm. In addition to a diuretic and an angiotensin-converting enzyme inhibitor, which of the following medicines should be taken by the patient?

A. Warfarin
B. Verapamil
C. Metoprolol
D. Doxazosin
E. L-dopa

CV

P 094 Which of the following is the primary pharmacologic effect of nitroglycerin?

A. Increase ventricular contractility
B. Decrease ventricular preload
C. Slow atrioventricular conduction
D. Increase afterload
E. Decrease slope 4 of sinoatrial action potential

CV, GU

P 095 Which of the following causes prolongation of the QT interval in a person's electrocardiogram?

A. Hypomagnesemia
B. Hyponatremia
C. Nitrate therapy
D. Angiotensin-converting enzyme inhibitor therapy
E. Hypercalcemia

NEURO

P 096 Presence of which of the following differentiates central cranial nerve VII palsy from peripheral cranial nerve VII palsy?

A. Ability to wrinkle forehead on affected side
B. Ability to close eye on affected side
C. Ataxia
D. Ability to taste on affected side
E. Nystagmus

CV, NEURO

P 097 A 12-year-old girl suddenly faints while playing soccer. Upon regaining consciousness, she is alert, pink, and asymptomatic. Blood pressure is 110/70 mm Hg; pulse, 80/min/regular; and respirations, 14/min. Cardiac, lung, and neurologic exam is normal. Which of the following is the most likely cause of the syncope?

A. Vasovagal faint
B. 3rd degree atrioventricular block
C. Long QT interval syndrome
D. Hypoglycemia
E. Hypertrophic obstructive cardiomyopathy

CV, PUL

P 098 A 47-year-old asthmatic woman suddenly has palpitations. Blood pressure is 110/70 mm Hg; pulse, 190/min/regular; and respirations, 20/min. Lung examination is normal. No murmur or gallop is heard. Electrocardiography shows paroxysmal supraventricular tachycardia. Which of the following is the preferred initial therapy?

A. Adenosine
B. Metoprolol
C. Digoxin
D. Verapamil
E. Ibutilide

GU

P 099 Which of the following is the most common complication of polycystic kidney disease?

A. Salt-losing nephropathy
B. Inappropriate ADH syndrome
C. Gout
D. Metabolic alkalosis
E. Hypertension

GU

P 100 Which of the following laboratory abnormalities is most suggestive of the diagnosis of acute glomerulonephritis?

A. White blood cell casts
B. Polyuria with fixed urine specific gravity
C. Oxalate crystals in urine
D. Red blood cell casts
E. Broad waxy casts in urine

ENDO, HEME

P 101 A 57-year-old woman has treated hypothyroidism for 4 years. Which of the following conditions is most likely to arise in this patient?

A. Interstitial nephritis
B. Pernicious anemia
C. Inappropriate ADH syndrome
D. Polycythemia rubra vera
E. Acute lymphoblastic leukemia

HEME, GI/N

P 102 A patient who has which of the following disorders will have gastric achlorhydria?

A. *Helicobacter pylori* gastric ulcer
B. Gastric lymphoma
C. Pernicious anemia
D. Achalasia of esophagus
E. Gastroparesis

HEME, GI/N

P 103 A patient who suffers from chronic alcohol abuse is most likely to show which of the following laboratory values?

A. Macrocytosis
B. Hypersegmented neutrophiles
C. Red blood cell casts in urine
D. Elevated serum thyrotropin level
E. Elevated plasma albumin level

ENDO

P 104 Presence of which of the following differentiates primary from secondary adrenal insufficiency?

A. Elevated plasma adrenocorticotropin level
B. Hypokalemia
C. Hypernatremia
D. Weight loss
E. Low plasma renin level

ENDO, CV

P 105 A 66-year-old man has a 2-month history of anorexia, a 7-pound weight loss, nausea, and generalized weakness. He now has dizziness upon arising from bed. In the sitting position, blood pressure is 90/70 mm Hg with pulse rate 76/min. Upon standing, blood pressure is 70/52 mm Hg with pulse rate 90/min. Which of the following is the most likely diagnosis?

   A. Primary hyperaldosteronism
   B. Adrenal insufficiency
   C. Carcinoid syndrome
   D. Pheochromocytoma
   E. Celiac disease

CV, DERM, HEME

P 106 A 34-year-old woman has the sudden onset of severe, constant anterior chest pain that is worsened by lying recumbent and eased by sitting and leaning forward. A malar rash is present. Which of the following laboratory values would be expected in this patient?

   A. Platelet count 450,000/microL
   B. Presence of serum anti-acetylcholine receptor antibodies
   C. White blood cell count 2000/microL
   D. Presence of serum anti-peroxidase antibodies
   E. White blood cell casts in urine

CV, DERM, HEME

P 107 A patient with systemic lupus erythematosus has a rash in the malar area and on the extremities. Which of the following is the appropriate counseling to be given to the patient?

   A. Apply coal tar and salicylate gel topically on weekly basis
   B. Avoid direct sunlight
   C. Avoid sunscreen preparations
   D. Take weekly cornstarch bath
   E. Avoid hydrocortisone topical medications

MS, CV

P 108 A 27-year-old woman has a 2-week history of diffuse joint aching. She now has the sudden onset of severe, persistent anterior chest pain. A pericardial friction rub is heard. Which of the following is the preferred diagnostic test in this patient?

   A. Serum C-reactive protein level
   B. 24-hour urinary 5-hydroxytryptamine excretion
   C. Presence of factor V Leiden
   D. 24-hour urinary calcium excretion
   E. Serum anti-nuclear antibody titer

EENT

P 109 A 37-year-old man has a recurrence of seasonal hay fever symptoms. Which of the following is the preferred treatment?

A. Intranasal phenylephrine
B. Intranasal beclomethasone
C. Oral chlorpheniramine
D. Oral cromolyn
E. Intranasal ipratropium

CV

P 110 In which of the following is a bicuspid aortic valve an associated congenital anomaly?

A. Patent ductus arteriosus
B. Coarctation of the aorta
C. Secundum atrial septal defect
D. Ebstein's anomaly
E. Polycystic kidney disease

CV, ID

P 111 A 6-year-old asymptomatic boy has a systolic ejection murmur and ejection click best heard near the apex. A bicuspid aortic valve is diagnosed. Which of the following is the most appropriate recommendation?

A. Avoid contact sports
B. Limit dietary calcium intake to 300 mg/day
C. Take daily penicillin G until age 12 years
D. No need for endocarditis prophylaxis
E. Have annual echocardiographic study

CV

P 112 A 40-year-old woman has recurrent chest pain that awakens her in the early morning hours. Variant angina pectoris is diagnosed. Which of the following is the preferred therapy?

A. Streptokinase
B. Aspirin
C. Metoprolol
D. Simvastatin
E. Verapamil

CV, ENDO

P 113 A 72-year-old man with hyperlipidemia has a 2-week history of exertional dyspnea without associated cough, chest discomfort, palpitations, or peripheral edema. Pulmonary function tests and chest radiography are normal. Which of the following is the preferred diagnostic test?

A. Outpatient cardiac monitoring
B. Thallium stress cardiac testing
C. Bronchoscopy
D. MRI scan of the chest
E. Serum brain natriuretic peptide level

HEME, CV

P 114 Which of the following is most likely to be associated with development of superior vena cava syndrome?

A. Non-Hodgkin's lymphoma
B. Squamous cell carcinoma of the lung
C. Thymoma
D. Adenocarcinoma of the pharynx
E. Medullary carcinoma of the thyroid

NEURO

P 115 Ability to perform which of the following is a test of cranial nerve V function?

A. Close eyes tightly
B. Raise shoulders against resistance
C. Smile
D. Move chin from side to side
E. Move eyes to lateral gaze

MS, GI/N

P 116 A 71-year-old man has elevation of serum alkaline phosphatase but normal serum gamma-glutamyl transpeptidase (GGTP) and normal serum calcium. Which of the following is the most likely diagnosis?

A. Pancreatic carcinoma
B. Paget's disease of bone
C. Chronic active hepatitis
D. Hyperparathyroidism
E. Metastatic tumor in the liver

CV

P 117 A 25-year-old asymptomatic man has a congenital bicuspid aortic valve. Which of the following is the most appropriate counseling for this patient?

A. Endocarditis prophylaxis is indicated
B. Significant aortic stenosis is likely to occur in adulthood
C. 80% likelihood of his children having bicuspid aortic valve
D. Take daily oral penicillin G, 125 mg
E. Undergo genetic typing

CV, PUL

P 118 A patient with chronic obstructive lung disease now has atrial fibrillation. Which of the following is the preferred medicine to control the ventricular rate?

A. Esmolol
B. Metoprolol
C. Quinidine
D. Verapamil
E. Adenosine

Section 1 ■ **Performance Test**

CV

P 119 A patient who has diffuse atherosclerotic vascular disease and claudication of the legs now has atrial fibrillation. Which of the following is the preferred medicine to control the ventricular rate?

A. Diltiazem
B. Metoprolol
C. Nifedipine
D. Sotalol
E. Propafenone

MS

P 120 A 72-year-old man is incidentally found on radiography of the hip to have Paget's disease of bone. Which of the following is the expected laboratory value?

A. Hypercalcemia
B. Elevated urinary hydroxyproline
C. Elevated serum gamma-glutamyl transpeptidase
D. Normal serum alkaline phosphatase
E. Elevated serum aminotransferase

CV

P 121 A 73-year-old man has chronic atrial fibrillation for which he takes digoxin and warfarin. His ventricular rate is poorly controlled, with ventricular rates always greater than 100/min. Which of the following is the most likely complication?

A. Dilated cardiomyopathy
B. 3rd degree atrioventricular block
C. Superior vena cava syndrome
D. Left atrial thrombus formation
E. Pulmonary infarction

GI/N

P 122 A 60-year-old man with cirrhosis and portal hypertension has an acute hemorrhage from ruptured esophageal varices. Which of the following is the preferred medicine to prevent recurrent bleeding?

A. Octreotide
B. Esomeprazole
C. Nadolol
D. Spironolactone
E. Nifedipine

GI/N

P 123 A 56-year-old man has cirrhosis due to chronic alcohol abuse. Serial measurement of which of the following serum levels would be most predictive of development of hepatocellular carcinoma?

A. Gamma-glutamyl transpeptidase
B. C-reactive protein
C. CA 125
D. Alpha-fetoprotein
E. Alkaline phosphatase

CV

P 124 A 44-year-old woman is diagnosed with variant angina. Which of the following is the expected finding on electrocardiography performed while the patient is having anginal discomfort?

A. ST segment depression
B. ST segment elevation
C. Isoelectric ST segments with T wave inversion
D. Widening of the QRS segments
E. Prolongation of the QT interval

ENDO, CV

P 125 A 32-year-old woman with diabetes mellitus is to begin angiotensin-converting enzyme inhibitor therapy for hypertension. Which of the following is the proper advice for this patient?

A. Do not become pregnant while on therapy
B. Do not take oral contraceptives while on therapy
C. Therapy increases the likelihood of twinning
D. Ensure daily intake of calcium >1000 mg/day
E. Use salt substitute for flavoring of food

DERM

P 126 Which of the following is most suggestive of the diagnosis of psoriasis?

A. Symmetrical arthritis
B. Pitting of nails
C. Maculopapular eruption
D. Clubbing of fingers and toes
E. Raynaud's phenomenon

PSY/LE

P 127 A 24-year-old woman has had three episodes of sudden, intense fear associated with trembling, palpitations, and dyspnea. These have each lasted 10 to 15 minutes. Each occurred a few days before normal menses. Which of the following is the most likely diagnosis?

A. Dissociative disorder
B. Panic disorder
C. Hypoglycemia
D. Pheochromocytoma
E. Carcinoid syndrome

CV

P 128 Which of the following is the proper advice to be given to a patient who is starting clonidine therapy for hypertension?

A. Take medication with milk or antacid
B. Do not take aspirin while on therapy
C. Red meat ingestion lessens efficacy of medication
D. Medication raises blood sugar
E. Withdraw medication over 1 week if it is to be discontinued

MS

P 129 Presence of which of the following differentiates psoriatic arthritis from rheumatoid arthritis on radiographic imaging?

A. Joint swelling
B. Demineralization
C. Joint space narrowing
D. "Sharpened pencil" appearance of fingers
E. Cartilaginous calcification

CV

P 130 A 72-year-old asymptomatic man with a history of remote myocardial infarction has new-onset hypertension. Left ventricular ejection fraction is 52%. Which of the following is the preferred initial class of medication for hypertensive therapy?

A. Angiotensin-converting enzyme inhibitor
B. Alpha 1-adrenergic blocker
C. Loop diuretic
D. Nondihydropine calcium channel blocker
E. Alpha 2a-adrenergic agonist

ENDO, CV

P 131 A 78-year-old woman with type 1 diabetes mellitus develops hypertension. Which of the following is the preferred initial medication in hypertensive therapy?

A. Verapamil
B. Doxazosin
C. Captopril
D. Losartan
E. Clonidine

DERM

P 132 A 37-year-old woman has ringworm on her trunk Which of the following is not a recommended therapy?

A. Betamethasone with clotrimazole (Lotrisone)
B. Miconazole (Lotrimin)
C. Econazole (Spectazole)
D. Butenafine (Mentax)
E. Terbinafine (Lamisil)

CV

P 133 A 42-year-old healthy woman has new-onset hypertension. Which of the following is the preferred initial medication in hypertensive therapy?

A. Hydrochlorothiazide
B. Captopril
C. Doxazosin
D. Verapamil
E. Metoprolol

MS

P 134 A 61-year-old woman with osteoporosis has new-onset hypertension. Which of the following is the preferred initial medication in hypertensive therapy?

A. Captopril
B. Hydralazine
C. Diltiazem
D. Hydrochlorothiazide
E. Propranolol

CV

P 135 A 59-year-old asymptomatic man has new-onset hypertension. His hemoglobin is 14 g/dL; blood urea nitrogen, 12 mg/dL; serum creatinine, 0.9 mg/dL; and serum uric acid, 11 mg/dL. Which of the following classes of medication is contraindicated in this patient?

A. Angiotensin-converting enzyme inhibitor
B. Alpha 1-adrenergic blocker
C. Angiotensin-receptor blocker
D. Thiazide
E. Calcium channel blocker

ENDO

P 136 A 16-year-old man has type 1 diabetes mellitus. Elevated plasma levels of which of the following would be expected?

A. Insulin
B. Glucagon
C. Epinephrine
D. 5-hydroxytryptamine
E. Cholecystokinin

DERM

P 137 A 28-year-old woman has two round lesions on her left arm. Examination shows rings of erythema with an advancing scaling border and central clearing. Which of the following is the most appropriate initial diagnostic test?

A. Punch biopsy
B. Serologic test for syphilis
C. Antinuclear antibody titer
D. Potassium hydroxide preparation of scales
E. Culture and sensitivity of lesion scrapings

REPRO, GU

P 138 Which of the following classes of medicine may cause sexual dysfunction in the male patient?

A. Selective serotonin receptor inhibitors
B. Angiotensin-converting enzyme inhibitors
C. Dihydropyridine calcium channel blockers
D. H2 receptor blockers
E. Carbonic anhydrase inhibitors

CV, GU

P 139 A 66-year-old man has had erectile dysfunction for 2 years. He now has stable angina pectoris for which he is taking aspirin, metoprolol, and isosorbide dinitrate. He should be advised to avoid which of the following?

A. H2 receptor blockers
B. Proton pump inhibitors
C. Herpes zoster immunization
D. Selenium hair compounds
E. Phosphodiesterase 5 inhibitors

DERM

P 140 A 24-year-old man is diagnosed as having scabies. Which of the following is the proper advice for the patient?

A. Washed clothing should be dried on hangers
B. Place clothes worn before diagnosis in plastic bag for 10 days
C. Spray recently worn clothes with peroxide
D. Destroy clothing worn for 10 days before diagnosis
E. Wear only white cotton clothing in contact with rash for 1 week

ID

P 141 A 16-year-old man has confirmed infectious mononucleosis. However, he does not get symptomatic relief of his sore throat using saline gargles and ibuprofen. A superimposed infection with which of the following organisms is most likely?

A. Cytomegalovirus
B. HHV-6
C. *Staphylococcus*
D. *Candida*
E. *Streptococcus*

DERM

P 142 A 40-year-old woman has a painful mouth. Examination shows violaceous papules with white streaks. Which of the following is the most likely diagnosis?

A. Psoriasis
B. Rosacea
C. Lichen planus
D. Erythema multiforme
E. Candidiasis

DERM

P 143 A 33-year-old man has an exacerbation of facial roseola. Which of the following is the recommended topical therapy?

A. Triamcinolone cream
B. Nystatin cream
C. Metronidazole gel
D. Miconazole cream
E. Clotrimazole cream

ID

P 144 An 18-year-old man has just recovered from infectious mononucleosis. Which of the following is proper counseling to be given to the patient?

A. Avoid aspirin intake for 3 months
B. May now participate in contact sports
C. Take daily supplement of glucosamine and chondroitin sulfate
D. Take daily supplement of creatine
E. Saliva may remain contagious for 6 months

DERM

P 145 Which of the following will worsen the rash of rosacea?

A. Milk ingestion
B. Alcohol ingestion
C. Angiotensin-converting enzyme inhibitor therapy
D. Alpha-adrenergic blocker therapy
E. St. John's wort ingestion

PUL, CV

P 146 A 56-year-old man with a 60 pack-year history of cigarette smoking has a 2-week history of worsening cough and dyspnea followed by the onset of abdominal distention and ankle swelling. Examination shows central cyanosis, elevated central venous pressure, scattered rhonchi, ascites, and peripheral edema. Which of the following is the most likely diagnosis?

A. Primary pulmonary hypertension
B. Cor pulmonale
C. Legionnaires' disease
D. Atrial septal defect
E. Eisenmenger's syndrome

CV, NEURO

P 147 A 77-year-old woman with hypertension and angina pectoris has a syncopal episode. Blood pressure is 84/60 mm Hg; pulse, 48/min/irregular; and respiratory rate, 19/min. Electrocardiography shows Mobitz I atrioventricular block. Which of the following is the most likely etiology of the syncopal episode?

A. Aspirin
B. Hydrochlorothiazide
C. Verapamil
D. Captopril
E. Isosorbide dinitrate

PUL, CV

P 148 A 49-year-old massively obese man has progressively worsening somnolence. Exam shows central cyanosis, elevated central venous pressure, and peripheral edema. Which of the following would be the expected systemic arterial blood gas values?

A. Pao_2 90 mm Hg, $Paco_2$ 40 mm Hg
B. Pao_2 60 mm Hg, $Paco_2$ 60 mm Hg
C. Pao_2 98 mm Hg, $Paco_2$ 60 mm Hg
D. Pao_2 90 mm Hg, $Paco_2$ 27 mm Hg
E. Pao_2 65 mm Hg, $Paco_2$ 30 mm Hg

ID, CV

P 149 For which of the following cardiac conditions is endocarditis prophylaxis not recommended?

A. Bioprosthetic heart valve
B. Tetralogy of Fallot
C. Mitral regurgitation in transplanted heart
D. Prior history of endocarditis
E. Mitral valve prolapse

PSY/LE

P 150 Sertraline (Zoloft) therapy is initiated in a 34-year-old woman for treatment of depression. She should be advised to avoid intake of which of the following?

A. Omega-3 fish oil
B. Aluminum-containing antacids
C. Spinach
D. St. John's wort
E. Ginseng

PSY/LE, NEURO

P 151 A 40-year-old man is transported to the emergency department. He is confused, constantly moving on the examining table, and exhibits spasmodic contractions of the facial and neck muscles. An adverse effect to which of the following is most likely?

A. Diazepam
B. Chlorpheniramine
C. Haloperidol
D. Ibuprofen
E. Nifedipine

CV

P 152 In a patient with newly diagnosed hypertension, a thiazide is preferred therapy over a nonselective beta-adrenergic blocker in a patient who has which of the following?

A. Cholelithiasis
B. Diverticulosis
C. Hyperthyroidism
D. Chronic obstructive lung disease
E. Chronic lymphocytic leukemia

GI/N

P 153 A 72-year-old woman with known diverticulosis has acute left lower quadrant abdominal pain, fever, and vomiting. Blood pressure is 78/60 mm Hg; pulse, 134/min; and respirations, 28/min. Exam shows a rigid abdomen without bowel sounds. Radiography shows free air under the left hemidiaphragm. Arterial blood gas determination indicates metabolic acidosis. Which of the following is the preferred initial treatment?

A. Infusion of dextrose 5% in water
B. Administration of intravenous norepinephrine
C. Insertion of intra-arterial balloon pump
D. Infusion of 0.9% saline
E. Administration of intravenous isoproterenol

PSY/LE

P 154 A 42-year-old woman takes sertraline (Zoloft) for treatment of depression. For the past 2 days she has taken a sympathomimetic medication for treatment of an acute upper respiratory infection. She is now transported to the emergency department because of the acute onset of agitation, delirium, and diarrhea. Blood pressure is 200/120 mm Hg; pulse, 136/min; and respiration, 22/min. Examination shows delirium, dilation of the pupils, flushed skin, and bilateral extensor Babinski signs. Which of the following is the most likely diagnosis?

A. Delirium tremens
B. Serotonin syndrome
C. Disorganized schizophrenia
D. Pheochromocytoma
E. Acute intermittent porphyria

ENDO

P 155 Which of the following is the primary pathophysiologic abnormality in type 1 diabetes mellitus?

A. Defect in compensatory insulin secretion
B. Defect in small bowel absorption of carbohydrate
C. Defect in urinary excretion of ketones
D. Exaggerated hepatic gluconeogenesis
E. Autoimmune destruction of pancreatic B cells

Section 1 ■ **Performance Test**

MS, CV

P 156 Indomethacin therapy is initiated in a 59-year-old man for treatment of hip osteoarthritis. He takes hydrochlorothiazide for hypertension. Which of the following is the most appropriate advice to be given to the patient?

A. Check serum sodium in 10 to 14 days
B. Check blood pressure in 10 to 14 days
C. Avoid ingestion of milk products while taking indomethacin
D. Avoid salt substitute
E. Take oral magnesium supplements

CV, GU

P 157 A 79-year-old man has systolic hypertension for which he takes hydrochlorothiazide. A recent blood urea nitrogen is 34 mg/dL and serum creatinine is 1.6 mg/dL. He should be advised to avoid which of the following?

A. Omega-3 fish oil
B. Ginseng
C. Chlorpheniramine
D. Cimetidine
E. Indomethacin

MS

P 158 Methotrexate therapy is to be initiated by a 47-year-old woman for treatment of rheumatoid arthritis. The patient should be advised to do which of the following?

A. Have liver function tests performed every 4 to 8 weeks
B. Have thyroid function tests performed every 4 months
C. Have annual bone marrow examination performed
D. Eat a high-purine diet
E. Avoid intake of magnesium-containing antacids

ENDO, MS

P 159 An 81-year-old woman has dyslipidemia for which she takes simvastatin. She is now advised to take acetaminophen for treatment of painful osteoarthritis of her knees and fingers. Which of the following is proper counseling for the patient?

A. Do not take acetaminophen in dosage > 2.0 g/day
B. Acetaminophen must be taken with food
C. Acetaminophen and simvastatin must be ingested at least 4 hours apart
D. Stop acetaminophen if warfarin therapy is advised in the future
E. Reduce simvastatin dosage to half of previously prescribed dosage

ID, CV

P 160 Endocarditis prophylaxis is recommended in a patient who has which of the following?

A. Mechanical heart valve in aortic position
B. Bicuspid aortic valve
C. Mitral valve prolapse with regurgitation
D. Rheumatic mitral valve stenosis
E. Hypertrophic obstructive cardiomyopathy

MS

P 161 A 62-year-old man has had recurrent attacks of acute gout. Which of the following is the primary factor that determines whether probenecid or allopurinol should be prescribed for the patient?

A. Level of 24-hour urinary excretion of uric acid
B. Level of serum uric acid
C. Urinary pH after overnight fast
D. Urinary osmolality after overnight fast
E. Level of 24-hour urinary protein excretion

CV, MS

P 162 A 59-year old man who takes hydrochlorothiazide for hypertension has just recovered from an attack of acute gout. Which of the following is proper counseling for the patient?

A. May continue hydrochlorothiazide therapy
B. Limit water intake to 24 ounces per day
C. May eat red meat and shellfish
D. Strictly limit intake of milk products
E. Avoid ingestion of alcohol

MS

P 163 During a physical examination, a healthy, asymptomatic 57-year-old man is found to have a serum uric acid of 9.0 mg/dL. He has never had an attack of gout. Which of the following is the most appropriate management?

A. Initiate allopurinol therapy
B. Initiate probenecid therapy
C. Limit intake of milk products
D. Reduce ingestion of red meat and shellfish
E. May drink beer; avoid hard spirits

CV

P 164 In a patient with newly-diagnosed hypertension, a thiazide diuretic is preferable to a beta-adrenergic blocker in a patient who has which of the following?

A. Angina pectoris
B. Leg claudication
C. Atrial fibrillation
D. Hyperuricemia
E. Acquired hemolytic anemia

REPRO, ENDO

P 165 Presence of which of the following differentiates polycystic ovary syndrome from metabolic syndrome?

A. Insulin resistance
B. Elevated serum estrogen
C. Reduced serum testosterone
D. Elevated serum luteinizing hormone
E. Low serum LDL cholesterol

ENDO

P 166 A 56-year-old woman has type 2 diabetes mellitus. Which of the following physical signs best correlates with insulin resistance in this patient?

A. Body mass index
B. Subcutaneous obesity
C. Leptin level in serum
D. Waist-to-hip fat ratio
E. Ankle brachial index

ENDO

P 167 A 34-year-old man has type 1 diabetes mellitus. Presence of which of the following would be an expected hematologic finding?

A. HLA-DR3 gene
B. Anti-Smith antibody
C. Anti-neutrophilic cytoplasm antibody
D. Elevated serum IgA level
E. Elevated erythrocyte sedimentation rate

GI/N, GU

P 168 On routine screening, an asymptomatic, vigorous man who takes no medication has a hemoglobin of 12 g/dL; blood urea nitrogen, 36 mg/dL; and serum creatinine of 0.9 mg/dL. Which of the following is the most appropriate test to be performed?

A. Creatinine clearance
B. Serum myoglobin level
C. 24-hour urinary sodium excretion
D. Stool for occult blood
E. 24-hour dietary protein intake measurement

GI/N, ENDO

P 169 A 24-year-old man has acute pancreatitis. He drinks no alcoholic beverages. Elevation in blood level of which of the following is most likely to be found in the patient?

A. Ferritin
B. Alpha-fetoprotein
C. Triglycerides
D. HDL cholesterol
E. Anti-phospholipid antibodies

GI, REPRO

P 170 A normal serum amylase level is most likely to be noted in a patient who has which of the following?

A. Mumps
B. Ruptured ectopic pregnancy
C. Renal failure
D. Diverticulosis
E. Pancreatic adenocarcinoma

PUL

P 171 A 4-year-old girl has had a common cold for 5 days. She now has fever, nonproductive cough, and chest soreness. Examination shows a noncyanotic, nontoxic patient with scattered rhonchi in both lung fields. Chest radiography shows an infiltrate consistent with pneumonia. Which of the following is the preferred therapy?

A. Doxycycline
B. Azithromycin
C. No antibiotic therapy
D. Penicillin G
E. Cephalexin

GI/N

P 172 An 18-year-old woman has protracted, severe diarrhea from enteritis. Which of the following is the best indicator of hypovolemia?

A. Serum sodium level
B. Urine specific gravity
C. Central venous pressure
D. Orthostatic hypotension
E. Resting heart rate

PSY/LE

P 173 A 20-year-old man is diagnosed as having panic disorder manifest by terror and chest pressure. Which of the following is the preferred urgent treatment of an episode?

A. Sublingual nitroglycerin
B. Oral temazepam (Restoril)
C. Oral hydroxyzine (Vistaril)
D. Oral phenobarbital
E. Sublingual lorazepam (Ativan)

GI/N, CV

P 174 A 56-year-old man with a history of alcohol abuse now has acute, severe pancreatitis. Blood pressure is 76/50 mm Hg; pulse, 140/min; and respirations, 30/min. Which of the following is the preferred initial intravenous therapy of the hemodynamic state?

A. Dopamine
B. Normal saline
C. Dextrose 5% in half-normal saline
D. Half-normal saline
E. Dextrose 2 ½% in half-normal saline

PUL, CV

P 175 One week after trauma to the left calf, a 56-year-old man has dyspnea without pleuritic chest pain or hemoptysis. Which of the following would make the diagnosis of pulmonary embolism very unlikely?

A. Normal oxygen saturation on pulse oximetry
B. Normal respiratory rate
C. Plasma fibrinogen level of 200 mg/mL
D. Normal systemic arterial pCO2 (Pa_{CO_2})
E. Serum D-dimer level of 400 nanogram/mL

ENDO, CV

P 176 Angiotensin-converting enzyme inhibitor (ACEI) therapy is initiated in a 34-year-old woman with type 1 diabetes mellitus for new-onset hypertension. Plasma blood urea nitrogen and serum creatinine levels are normal. Which of the following is appropriate counseling to the patient?

A. Angioedema typically occurs after 4 months of therapy
B. Take the medication with milk
C. Avoid nonselective nonsteroidal anti-inflammatory medicines
D. ACEI therapy increases risk of developing atrial fibrillation
E. Avoid pregnancy

CV

P 177 A 34-year-old obese man has a 3-day history of left calf soreness. Examination shows no overlying erythema or palpable venous cord in the calf. Which of the following would signify that a duplex ultrasound study may be omitted from the diagnostic plan?

A. Negative Homans' sign
B. Lack of calf edema
C. Serum D-dimer level of 400 ng/mL
D. Equal skin temperature in both calves
E. Erythrocyte sedimentation rate of 20 mm/hr

CV

P 178 A 78-year-old man has an acute ST segment elevation acute anterior wall myocardial infarction (STEMI). Blood pressure is 130/70 mm Hg; pulse, 90/min; and respirations, 21/min. There is no clinical evidence of heart failure. In addition to nitroglycerin, aspirin, and alteplase, which of the following medicines should be given to the patient?

A. Clopidogrel
B. Tirofiban (Aggrastat)
C. Intravenous nitroprusside
D. Captopril
E. Digoxin

ID, PUL

P 179 A 39-year-old man in excellent health has a 2-day history of fever to 102°F, productive cough, and chest soreness. Blood pressure is 120/70 mm Hg; pulse, 112/min; and respirations, 22/min. Exam shows dullness to percussion and bronchial breath sounds at the right lung base. Which of the following is the preferred therapy?

A. Admit for intravenous penicillin therapy
B. Outpatient treatment with penicillin G
C. Outpatient treatment with clarithromycin
D. Admit for intravenous macrolide therapy
E. Obtain sputum and blood cultures; await results before starting antibiotic

ID, PUL

P 180 A 28-year-old man with cystic fibrosis has a 3-day history of fever and productive cough. Chest radiography shows right lower lobe pneumonia with a small cavity containing fluid. Which of the following is the most likely infecting organism?

A. *Klebsiella pneumoniae*
B. Respiratory syncytial virus
C. *Chlamydia pneumoniae*
D. *Streptococcus pneumoniae*
E. *Pseudomonas aeruginosa*

PUL, CV

P 181 A 42-year-old woman who has allergic asthma now has new-onset hypertension. Angiotensin-converting enzyme inhibitor (ACEI) therapy is being considered. Which of the following is the most appropriate clinical statement about ACEI therapy in this patient?

A. Increased likelihood of ACEI causing cough
B. Increased likelihood of exacerbating airflow obstruction
C. Diminished anti-hypertensive effect due to underlying asthma
D. Tolerated as well as in nonasthmatic
E. Increased likelihood of causing hyperkalemia

ID, PUL

P 182 A localized outbreak of Legionnaires' disease has been identified. Which of the following is the most likely source?

A. Contaminated food in a restaurant
B. Sick cows on a local farm
C. Cough aerosols from sick colleagues
D. Hotel showers
E. Malfunction in community sanitation system

PUL, ID

P 183 A 72-year-old woman with chronic obstructive lung disease has a 4-day history of fever and productive cough. One week earlier, she had returned from a vacation resort where she had used the hot tubs on a daily basis. Examination shows the patient to be acutely ill with decreased breath sounds at the left lung base. Chest radiography demonstrates pneumonia with lung abscess. Which of the following is the most likely diagnosis?

A. Pneumococcal pneumonia
B. Anthrax pneumonia
C. Chlamydial pneumonia
D. Legionnaires' disease
E. Psittacosis

CV, GI/N

P 184 A 64-year-old obese man has hypertension and remote history of myocardial infarction. Which of the following foods would not be considered part of a prudent diet?

A. Partially hydrogenated coffee creamer
B. Peanuts
C. Salmon
D. Olive oil
E. Salt substitute

PUL, ID

P 185 A 41-year-old woman has a 2-day history of fever, cough productive of green sputum, and left pleuritic chest pain. Examination shows dullness to percussion, decreased tactile fremitus, and decreased breath sounds over the lower one third of the left posterior chest. Which of the following is the most likely diagnosis?

A. Atelectasis of the left lower lobe
B. Left hemothorax
C. Bronchogenic carcinoma
D. Bronchiectasis
E. Pneumonia with effusion

CV

P 186 An 83-year-old man with a long history of hypertension has severe, prolonged chest pain. Acute myocardial infarction is diagnosed. Blood pressure is 220/126 mm Hg; pulse, 102/min; and respirations, 20/min. Examination shows clear lung fields and apical S4 gallop without murmur. Which of the following is contraindicated at this time?

A. t-PA
B. Metoprolol
C. Clopidogrel
D. Nitroglycerin
E. Captopril

PUL, ENDO

P 187 A 62-year-old woman has small cell carcinoma complicated by inappropriate anti-diuretic hormone secretion (SIADH). Which of the following is the most likely laboratory abnormality to be noted?

   A. Elevated serum osmolality
   B. Pleural fluid glucose level of 120 mg/dL
   C. Systemic arterial pH of 7.47
   D. Hyperphosphatemia
   E. Hyponatremia

MS, GI/N

P 188 A 74-year-old man has severe osteoarthritis of the hips. In addition, he has chronic heartburn. The patient should be counseled that there may be an increased risk of which of the following when celecoxib (Celebrex) therapy is initiated?

   A. Seizures
   B. Myocardial infarction
   C. Hemolytic anemia
   D. Adult respiratory distress syndrome
   E. Paroxysmal atrial fibrillation

ENDO, GI/N

P 189 Despite studious efforts, a 63-year-old man with type 1 diabetes mellitus has repeated episodes of nausea, bloating, and wide swings in his plasma glucose levels. Which of the following is the most likely cause?

   A. Gastroparesis
   B. Malabsorption syndrome
   C. Insulin resistance syndrome
   D. Villous atrophy of small bowel
   E. Hepatocellular carcinoma

PUL, GI/N

P 190 A 61-year-old man who has which of the following diseases is most likely to have a transudative pleural effusion?

   A. Pneumococcal pneumonia
   B. Adenocarcinoma of the lung
   C. Pancreatitis
   D. Nephrotic syndrome
   E. Sarcoidosis

CV

P 191 A 76-year-old man has prolonged, severe anterior chest pressure. Extensive anterior myocardial infarction is diagnosed. The patient has a history of cerebral hemorrhage 4 years earlier. Blood pressure is 130/70 mm Hg; pulse, 100/min; and respirations, 20/min. There is no clinical evidence of heart failure. Which of the following is contraindicated?

A. Oral aspirin
B. Intravenous metoprolol
C. Intravenous nitroglycerin
D. Oral captopril
E. Intravenous alteplase

GI/N, ENDO

P 192 A 55-year-old woman who has type 1 diabetes mellitus is suspected of now having gastroparesis. Which of the following is the preferred diagnostic test?

A. Upper gastrointestinal endoscopy
B. Nuclear scintigraphy after radioactive-labeled meal
C. 24-hour esophageal pH monitoring
D. Upper gastrointestinal series with Gastrografin
E. CT imaging of the abdomen after overnight fast

GU, ID

P 193 A 15-year-old male has urethritis due to *Neisseria gonorrhoeae*. Which of the following is not recommended in the management of the patient?

A. Cefoxitin
B. Doxycycline
C. Ofloxacin
D. Spectinomycin
E. Azithromycin

DERM

P 194 A 56-year-old healthy man has a 1-day history of constant burning pain extending in a line from his back around to his right anterior chest. The pain does not increase with inspiration or bending. Examination of the skin, chest, lung, and heart is normal. The patient should be advised of which of the following?

A. Pleurodynia is most likely diagnosis
B. Bedrest for 48 hours is advised
C. Zoster rash may appear in 24 to 48 hours
D. Ventilation/perfusion scan is indicated
E. Serial cardiac enzyme determination is advised

GI/N

P 195 Which of the following determinations is most specific for defining portal hypertension as the cause of ascites in a patient?

A. Ascites fluid total protein level
B. Ascites fluid triglyceride level
C. Ascites fluid lactic dehydrogenase level
D. Serum to ascites albumin gradient
E. Ascites fluid glucose level

GI/N

P 196 A 62-year-old man with known cirrhosis complicated by portal hypertension and ascites has a 2-day history of fever and abdominal pain. Rectal temperature is 101°F; blood pressure, 90/72 mm Hg; pulse, 110/min; and respirations, 26/min. Examination shows ascites with diffuse abdominal tenderness. White blood cell count is 14,000/microL and systemic arterial blood gas reveals a pH of 7.21. Which of the following is the most likely diagnosis?

A. Carcinoma of pancreas
B. Cholecystitis
C. Mesenteric infarction
D. Spontaneous bacterial peritonitis
E. Angiodysplasia of the colon

ID, GI/N

P 197 Two days after returning from a mountain hiking trip, a 26-year-old man has profuse watery diarrhea, abdominal cramps, and nausea. No fever is present. Which of the following is the most likely infectious organism?

A. Enterotoxigenic *Escherichia coli*
B. *Campylobacter jejuni*
C. Rotavirus
D. *Giardia lamblia*
E. Adenovirus

ID, GI/N

P 198 In a healthy patient, presence of which of the following differentiates enteritis due to *Campylobacter jejuni* from *Giardia lamblia*?

A. Axillary temperature of 103.6°F
B. Incubation period of 3 weeks
C. Association with noninfectious urethritis
D. Fecal presence of leukocytes
E. Fecal presence of eosinophiles

GI/N, ID

P 199 A 3-year-old girl who has been swimming in a community pool has the sudden onset of watery diarrhea and infrequent vomiting. Which of the following is the most likely infecting organism?

A. Rotavirus
B. Norovirus
C. Cytomegalovirus
D. Enterotoxigenic *Escherichia coli*
E. *Cryptosporidium*

ID, GI/N

P 200 A 61-year-old man with which of the following underlying conditions should take antimicrobial prophylaxis to prevent traveler's diarrhea?

A. History of remote myocardial infarction
B. Irritable bowel syndrome
C. Diabetes insipidus
D. Paroxysmal atrial fibrillation
E. Idiopathic pulmonary fibrosis

CV, ID

P 201 A 71-year-old woman has an indwelling intravenous catheter in her right forearm. She has a 1-day history of aching pain and redness in that arm. Oral temperature 98.6°F. Examination shows induration, erythema, and a tender venous cord in the right forearm. White blood cell count is 9800/microL. In addition to catheter removal, which of the following is the preferred therapy?

A. Unfractionated heparin
B. Application of cold compresses to affected area
C. Low molecular weight heparin
D. Nafcillin
E. Splinting of right forearm and wrist

CV

P 202 A 36-year-old man has a 3-week history of worsening dyspnea without cough or wheezing. Three years earlier he was shot in the right thigh. Blood pressure is 164/56 mm Hg; pulse, 121/min; and respirations, 30/min. Examination shows bounding pulses, bibasilar rales, and apical S3 gallop. A thrill is felt over the scar in the right thigh. Which of the following is the most likely diagnosis?

A. Hyperthyroidism
B. Beriberi
C. Paget's disease of bone
D. Iron deficiency anemia
E. Arteriovenous fistula

ID, ENDO, REPRO

P 203 Live, attenuated influenza vaccine is recommended for which of the following persons?

A. Healthy 22-year-old nurse
B. Patient with diabetes mellitus
C. Pregnant woman
D. Heart failure patient
E. Nephrotic syndrome patient

ENDO, HEME

P 204 Propylthiouracil therapy is initiated for a 40-year-old woman who has Graves' disease. Onset of which of the following is considered to be associated with agranulocytosis?

A. Insomnia
B. Palpitations
C. Headache
D. Puffiness of fingers
E. Sore throat

CV, ENDO

P 205 A 28-year-old woman has a 2-week history of dyspnea and bilateral ankle edema. Blood pressure is 166/58 mm Hg; pulse, 126/min; and respirations, 26/min. Examination shows warm skin, lid lag, bounding pulses, bibasilar rales, and fine tremor. Which of the following is the most likely diagnosis?

A. Myasthenia gravis
B. Essential tremor
C. Mercury poisoning
D. Hyperthyroidism
E. Arteriovenous fistula

GI/N

P 206 Which of the following classes of medication may produce acute bloody diarrhea due to an inflammatory colitis?

A. Nonaspirin, nonselective, nonsteroidal anti-inflammatory
B. Angiotensin-converting enzyme inhibitor
C. Calcium channel blocker
D. Thyroid hormone
E. Thiazide

GU

P 207 A 34-year-old man has metabolic acidosis of indeterminate cause. The anion gap equals which of the following?

A. $Na - (Cl + HCO_3 + albumin)$
B. $(Na + K + Mg) - (Cl + HCO_3)$
C. $pCO2$ in mm Hg $- HCO_3$ in mEq/L
D. $Na - (Cl + HCO_3)$
E. $(Na + K) - (Cl + HCO_3 + lactate)$

ID

P 208 Trivalent inactivated influenza vaccine is not recommended for which of the following patients?

A. 47-year-old healthy woman
B. Chronic obstructive lung disease patient
C. Heart failure patient
D. Hemoglobinopathy patient
E. Patient taking chronic warfarin therapy

NEURO

P 209 A 34-year-old woman has the sudden onset of an intensely severe headache followed quickly by nausea and vomiting. Vital signs are normal. Examination shows nuchal rigidity. CT imaging of the brain is normal. Which of the following is the most appropriate next diagnostic test for suspected subarachnoid hemorrhage?

A. Cerebral angiography
B. Magnetic resonance angiography
C. MRI scan of the brain
D. Lumbar puncture
E. Electroencephalogram

NEURO

P 210 Twenty-four hours after a lumbar puncture, a 34-year-old woman has a persistent frontal headache. This is unresponsive to bedrest and oral analgesics. Administration of which of the following is the next preferred treatment?

A. Intramuscular adrenocorticotrophic hormone
B. Oral caffeine
C. Intramuscular methylprednisolone
D. Epidural blood patch
E. Intramuscular morphine sulfate

REPRO, NEURO

P 211 A 28-year-old woman, in her 35th week of pregnancy, has recurrent pain and tingling in the first and second fingers of both hands. Symptoms are worse at night. Tinel's sign is positive. Which of the following is recommended management?

A. Indomethacin for 2 weeks
B. Corticosteroid injection into the carpal tunnel
C. Surgical decompression of the carpal tunnel
D. Electrophysiologic study of the median nerves
E. Assurance to patient that symptoms disappear after delivery

GI/N

P 212 A 24-year-old woman has diarrhea with gross rectal bleeding. She is diagnosed as having ulcerative colitis limited to the proctosigmoid area. Which of the following is the preferred therapy?

A. Oral sulfasalazine
B. 2-week course of tapering glucocorticoids
C. 1-week course of oral infliximab
D. Hydrocortisone foam enemas
E. Oral clindamycin

ENDO

P 213 A 49-year-old woman has newly diagnosed Graves' disease. Presence of which of the following in the blood is most specific to confirm this diagnosis?

A. Anti-thyroglobulin antibodies
B. Th1 CD4+ lymphocytes
C. Anti–thyroid-stimulating hormone receptor antibodies
D. Anti-thyroid peroxidase antibodies
E. HLA-antigen complex

ID, GU

P 214 A 76-year-old woman is in septic shock due to gram-negative bacteremia. An increase in which of the following is the pathophysiologic basis for the metabolic acidosis that is present?

A. Loss of bicarbonate in stool
B. Production of lactic acid
C. Loss of bicarbonate in urine
D. Production of ketone bodies
E. Production of ammonia

GI/N

P 215 A 34-year-old man has a 1-week history of recurrent bloody diarrhea and fecal urgency. He has taken no medication for 6 months and has not traveled outside the United States for 3 years. Which of the following is the preferred initial diagnostic test?

A. Flexible sigmoidoscopy
B. Barium enema
C. CT imaging of the colon
D. Mesenteric angiography
E. Stool assay for *Clostridium difficile* toxin

NEURO, ENDO

P 216 Over a period of 1 month, a 62-year-old woman has developed bilateral carpal tunnel syndrome. Which of the following is the preferred diagnostic test?

A. Serum C-reactive protein
B. Erythrocyte sedimentation rate
C. Serum anti-nuclear antibody titer
D. Serum thyroid-stimulating hormone level
E. Serum anti-Sm antibody titer

GI/N

P 217 A 42-year-old man with gastroesophageal reflux should be advised to avoid which of the following?

A. Blueberries
B. Rice pudding
C. Bread pudding
D. Raspberry sherbet
E. Chocolate ice cream

GU, ENDO

P 218 A patient has end-stage renal disease due to diabetic nephropathy. Which of the following acid-base conditions would most likely be present?

A. Increased anion gap metabolic acidosis
B. Metabolic alkalosis
C. Respiratory acidosis
D. Normal systemic arterial pH
E. Normal anion gap metabolic acidosis

CV, ENDO

P 219 A 72-year-old woman with known coronary artery disease has newly diagnosed hyperthyroidism due to a toxic adenoma of the thyroid. Which of the following is recommended therapy prior to administration of radioactive iodine?

A. Iodine
B. Thyroglobulin
C. Prednisone
D. Methimazole
E. Doxazosin

GI/N

P 220 A 62-year-old obese woman has a 3-week history of recurrent heartburn occurring, on average, twice each week. The symptoms are present only at night, awakening the patient approximately 3 hours after retiring. Which of the following is the preferred initial therapy?

A. Calcium carbonate at bedtime
B. Aluminum hydroxide/magnesium carbonate/alginate at bedtime
C. Omeprazole before breakfast and dinner
D. Ranitidine at bedtime
E. Omeprazole and cimetidine before breakfast

ENDO

P 221 Which of the following is considered to be the most sensitive test for the diagnosis of hyperthyroidism due to a toxic adenoma of the thyroid?

A. Serum T3 level
B. Serum thyroid-stimulating hormone level
C. T3 resin uptake
D. Free T4 index
E. Thyroid hormone binding ratio

GI/N

P 222 Which of the following is a potential long-term complication in the ulcerative colitis patient who has extensive colon involvement?

A. Aseptic necrosis of the femur
B. Colon cancer
C. Angiodysplasia of the colon
D. Gangrene of the colon
E. Toxic megacolon

EENT, GI/N

P 223 A 56-year-old obese man who has never smoked now has a 4-week history of hoarseness. He has no heartburn or dysphagia. He takes no medication. Which of the following is the most likely cause?

A. Zenker's diverticulum
B. Squamous cell carcinoma of esophagus
C. Postnasal drip
D. Epiglottitis
E. Gastroesophageal reflux

REPRO, CV

P 224 Presence of which of the following differentiates preeclampsia from gestational hypertension?

A. Fasting plasma glucose >140 mg/dL
B. Proteinuria
C. Patient was normotensive prior to pregnancy
D. Onset of hypertension at 12th to 16th week of gestation
E. Recognized association with migraine headaches

REPRO

P 225 Presence of which of the following differentiates eclampsia from preeclampsia?

A. Hypertension
B. Proteinuria
C. Thrombocytopenia
D. Blurred vision
E. Seizures

REPRO

P 226 A 33-year-old woman is diagnosed as having antiphospholipid antibody syndrome. Which of the following is the most likely complication to occur in the patient if she were pregnant?

A. Subarachnoid hemorrhage
B. Nephrotic syndrome
C. Placenta previa
D. Gestational diabetes
E. Recurrent fetal loss

REPRO

P 227 Which of the following is the primary pathophysiologic mechanism thought responsible for the development of preeclampsia?

A. Vasodilation of the placental arteries
B. Excess secretion of catecholamines
C. Endothelial dysfunction
D. Down regulation of adrenergic receptors
E. Increased secretion of brain natriuretic peptide

REPRO

P 228 Eight weeks after her last normal menstrual period, a 26-year-old woman has abdominal pain and vaginal bleeding. Which of the following diagnostic tests is preferred in order to differentiate between ectopic pregnancy and threatened abortion?

A. Serum hCG concentration
B. MRI scan of the pelvis
C. Serum progesterone level
D. Transvaginal ultrasonography
E. Fetal karyotype determination

REPRO

P 229 Which of the following is considered to be the highest risk factor for ectopic pregnancy?

A. Maternal age >35 years
B. Current cigarette smoking
C. History of bipolar coagulation sterilization
D. In vitro fertilization
E. Regular vaginal douching

ID, GI/N

P 230 A 27-year-old woman has the following hepatitis B serologic markers:

HBsAg positive

Anti-HBc negative

Anti-HBs positive

Which of the following is the clinical status of the patient?

A. Acute hepatitis B infection
B. Chronic hepatitis B infection
C. Susceptible to hepatitis B infection
D. Immune due to hepatitis B vaccination
E. Immune due to natural infection

GI/N, PSY/LE

P 231 A 49-year-old man has jaundice determined to be due to intrahepatic cholestasis. Which of the following medicines is most likely to be the causative agent?

A. Risperidone (Risperdal)
B. Paroxetine (Paxil)
C. Chlorpromazine (Thorazine)
D. Sertraline (Zoloft)
E. Nortriptyline (Pamelor)

HEME, GI/N

P 232 A 19-year-old woman has jaundice of the sclera and palms. Total serum bilirubin is 3.2 mg/dL, conjugated bilirubin is 0.4 mg/dL, and unconjugated fraction is 2.8 mg/dL. Serum alanine aminotransferase is 40 units/L and serum alkaline phosphatase is 45 units/L. Which of the following is the most likely diagnosis?

A. Hepatic sarcoidosis
B. Choledocholithiasis
C. Infectious mononucleosis
D. Systemic lupus erythematosus
E. Hemolytic anemia

GI/N, ID

P 233 A 57-year-old man has acute right upper quadrant abdominal pain radiating to his right shoulder, nausea, fever, and chills. Blood pressure is 104/70 mm Hg; pulse, 130/min; rectal temperature, 103°F. Examination shows scleral icterus and right upper quadrant abdominal tenderness without rebound. White blood cell count is 31,000/microL with left shift. Which of the following is the most likely diagnosis?

A. Acute cholecystitis
B. Primary sclerosing cholangitis
C. Primary biliary cirrhosis
D. Viral hepatitis
E. Ascending cholangitis

GI/N

P 234 A 47-year-old woman has a 3-week history of worsening fatigue and pruritus. Examination shows scleral icterus. Presence of which of the following serum antibodies is most specific for the diagnosis of primary biliary cirrhosis?

A. Anti-nuclear
B. Anti-Sm
C. Anti-smooth muscle
D. Anti-mitochondrial
E. Ant-actin

GI/N

P 235 A 63-year-old man has jaundice. Which of the following laboratory values is most suggestive of the diagnosis of alcoholic hepatitis?

A. Elevated serum globulins
B. Ratio of serum AST/ALT is >2:1
C. Hypoalbuminemia
D. Elevated serum cholesterol
E. Presence of serum anti-mitochondrial antibodies

GU

P 236 A 23-year-old woman has recurrent episodes of severe lower abdominal cramping that starts with the onset of menstrual bleeding. Primary dysmenorrhea is diagnosed. In addition to heat application to the abdomen, oral administration of which of the following is the preferred therapy?

A. Oxycodone
B. Ibuprofen
C. Magnesium
D. Nifedipine
E. Vitamin B_6

GU, PSY/LE

P 237 A 33-year-old woman has premenstrual dysphoric disorder manifest primarily by depression and hopelessness. Which of the following classes of medicine is the preferred therapy?

A. Benzodiazepine
B. Potassium-sparing diuretic
C. GnRH agonist
D. Androgen
E. Selective serotonin reuptake inhibitor

GU, ENDO, CV

P 238 A 76-year-old woman with a history of type 2 diabetes mellitus is hospitalized for treatment of lobar pneumonia. Twenty-four hours later, she has polyuria and polydipsia. Plasma glucose is 622 mg/dL and serum osmolality is 315 mOsmol/Kg. Which of the following is the least likely laboratory abnormality to be present?

  A. Anion gap of 18 mEq/L
  B. Systemic arterial pH 7.37
  C. Normal serum lactate concentration
  D. Serum potassium 3.9 mEq/L
  E. Serum bicarbonate 24 mEq/L

GU, ENDO

P 239 An obese 61-year-old man has type 2 diabetes mellitus. His serum creatinine concentration is 1.6 mEq/dL. Initiation of metformin therapy in this patient increases the risk for which of the following?

  A. Sodium-losing nephropathy
  B. Acute pericarditis
  C. Altered awareness of hypoglycemia
  D. "Dawn" phenomenon
  E. Lactic acidosis

ENDO, GI/N

P 240 A 57-year-old woman with which of the following should not receive metformin therapy for type 2 diabetes mellitus?

  A. Heavy alcohol intake
  B. Greater than 20% overweight
  C. Hypertension
  D. Left ventricular ejection fraction <40%
  E. Sensitivity to iodide contrast media

GU, ENDO

P 241 A 67-year-old man who is receiving metformin therapy for type 2 diabetes mellitus is to undergo peripheral arteriography utilizing a radiocontrast agent. Which of the following is proper counseling for the patient?

  A. NPO for 12 hours prior to imaging study
  B. Do not take metformin on morning of study
  C. Take furosemide 40 mg orally at 6 AM on day of study
  D. Take 20 mEq potassium chloride at 6 AM on day of study
  E. Switch to a sulfonylurea agent 1 week prior to study

EENT, PUL

P 242 A healthy 33-year-old man has a 3-day history of nasal congestion, rhinorrhea, sore throat, and cough productive of mucoid sputum. The patient has not had fever. Vital signs are normal. Examination shows nasal congestion and scattered bilateral wheezes. Which of the following medicines should not be prescribed?

A. Ipratropium
B. Ibuprofen
C. Aspirin
D. Azithromycin
E. Phenylephrine

CV

P 243 A 78-year-old man has an acute myocardial infarction complicated by recurrent runs of ventricular tachycardia. In the intensive care unit he becomes stuporous and confused. Vital signs are normal. Cardiac monitoring shows normal sinus rhythm. Which of the following medicines is the most likely cause of the mental change?

A. Streptokinase
B. Lidocaine
C. Aspirin
D. Metoprolol
E. Nitroglycerin

GU

P 244 A 57-year-old man with a history of chronic renal insufficiency has a serum potassium concentration of 6.5 mEq/L. Which of the following is the preferred initial therapy?

A. Subcutaneous administration of regular insulin
B. Retention enema of sodium polystyrene (Kayexalate)
C. Hemodialysis
D. Intravenous administration of verapamil
E. Administration of nebulized albuterol

CV, GI/N

P 245 A 51-year-old woman receives furosemide for treatment of portal hypertension with ascites. Which of the following on electrocardiography is most suggestive of hypokalemia?

A. Peaked T waves
B. Shortened QT interval
C. Mobitz I atrioventricular block
D. Flattening of T waves with prominent U waves
E. Absence of P waves with widening of QRS complex

NEURO

P 246 A patient who has myasthenia gravis would be expected to have which of the following serum antibodies?

A. Anti-acetylcholine
B. Anti-parietal cell
C. Anti-Sm
D. Anti–double-stranded DNA
E. Anti–smooth-muscle

ENDO

P 247 Presence of which of the following differentiates Graves' disease from hyperthyroidism due to a toxic thyroid nodule?

A. Atrial fibrillation
B. Decreased serum thyroid-stimulating hormone level
C. Lid lag
D. Increased cardiac output
E. Anti–thyroid-stimulating hormone antibodies

GU

P 248 A 42-year-old man has nephrotic syndrome due to focal glomerulosclerosis. In addition to sodium restriction and diuretic therapy, which of the following should be received by the patient?

A. Oral calcium channel blocker
B. Oral alpha-adrenergic blocker
C. Intermittent intravenous infusion of albumin
D. Oral COX-2 nonsteroidal anti-inflammatory agent
E. Oral angiotensin-converting enzyme inhibitor

CV, GU

P 249 A 47-year-old woman has nephrotic syndrome. Which of the following is the most likely complication to occur?

A. Subdural hematoma
B. Deep vein thrombosis
C. Chronic pyelonephritis
D. Spontaneous bacterial peritonitis
E. Avascular necrosis of the femur

HEME

P 250 A 20-year-old man has a 3-week history of dry cough and 1-week history of night sweats. Vital signs are normal. Examination shows enlarged right cervical, left inguinal, and left supraclavicular lymph nodes. No murmur or gallop is heard. Which of the following is the most likely diagnosis?

A. Endocarditis
B. Adverse reaction to retinoid therapy
C. Hodgkin's disease
D. Primary tuberculosis
E. Sarcoidosis

NEURO

P 251 Presence of which of the following differentiates essential tremor from Parkinson's disease?

A. Asymmetric pupil size
B. Drooling
C. Tremor of the lips
D. Normal gait
E. Orthostatic hypotension

NEURO

P 252 Presence of which of the following differentiates amyotrophic lateral sclerosis from Parkinson's disease?

A. Tremor
B. Orthostatic hypotension
C. Loss of sweating
D. Absence of deep tendon reflexes
E. Fasciculations

CV, EENT, NEURO

P 253 A 79-year-old woman has had three episodes, each lasting 5 to 10 minutes, of blurred vision in both eyes; dizziness; and unstable gait. Blood pressure in the right arm, sitting, is 150/80 mm Hg and in the left arm, sitting, 118/74 mm Hg. Neurologic examination performed when the patient is asymptomatic is normal. Which of the following is the most likely diagnosis?

A. Takayasu's arteritis
B. Coarctation of aorta
C. Giant cell arteritis
D. Subclavian steal syndrome
E. Thrombosis of left common carotid artery

NEURO, CV

P 254 Subclavian steal syndrome is diagnosed in an 82-year-old man who has left arm claudication. Which of the following is the preferred treatment?

A. Regional sympathetic nerve block
B. Administration of oral nifedipine
C. Administration of oral prednisone
D. Ventricular-atrial shunting procedure
E. Percutaneous luminal angioplasty

GU, ENDO

P 255 A 63-year-old woman with type 2 diabetes mellitus has nephrotic syndrome. In addition to sodium restriction and a diuretic, which of the following classes of medicine is appropriate therapy?

A. Glucocorticoid
B. Alpha-adrenergic blocker
C. Alkylating agent
D. Angiotensin-converting enzyme inhibitor
E. Interferon-alpha

REPRO

P 256   A 26-year-old woman wishes to become pregnant but is concerned because of a family history of sudden infant death syndrome (SIDS). Which of the following is the most important counseling for the patient with specific reference to SIDS?

A. Avoid gaining more than 16 pounds during pregnancy
B. Do not smoke during pregnancy
C. Have fasting blood sugar determination every 7 to 8 weeks during pregnancy
D. Fetal genetic typing should be performed during pregnancy
E. Patient should be checked for acyl-CoA dehydrogenase deficiency

NEURO, CV

P 257   Which of the following adverse effects is common to levodopa-carbidopa, dopamine agonists, and catecholamine-O-methyltransferase inhibitors used in therapy of Parkinson's disease?

A. Autoimmune hemolytic anemia
B. Colitis
C. Thrombocytosis
D. Atrioventricular block
E. Orthostatic hypotension

REPRO, GU

P 258   A 33-year-old woman who has which of the following conditions should preferably take a progestin-only contraceptive?

A. History of deep vein thrombosis
B. Post partum >21 days and not breastfeeding
C. Obesity
D. Epilepsy
E. HIV infected

ENDO, REPRO

P 259   A 36-year-old pregnant woman has gestational diabetes mellitus. A cardiovascular fitness program has resulted in normalization of her glucose tolerance. Which of the following is the primary physiologic mechanism by which exercise improves glucose control?

A. Increases tissue sensitivity to insulin
B. Decreases hepatic gluconeogenesis
C. Decreases glycogenolysis
D. Reduces cellular oxidative stress
E. Increases acetyl Co-A protein

REPRO, ENDO

P 260 A 34-year-old woman who takes a single dose of glyburide daily for treatment of type 2 diabetes mellitus wishes to become pregnant. Which of the following is the most appropriate counseling for the patient when she becomes pregnant?

A. Glyburide should be taken twice daily
B. Morning insulin therapy should be added to the glyburide
C. A trial period of nonhypoglycemic treatment should be attempted
D. Glyburide should be replaced by metformin therapy
E. Glyburide therapy must be replaced by insulin

HEME

P 261 Presence of which of the following differentiates intravascular hemolysis from extravascular hemolysis?

A. Hemosiderinuria
B. Elevation of serum indirect bilirubin
C. Absent serum haptoglobin
D. Hypersegmented neutrophils on peripheral smear examination
E. Nucleated red blood cells on peripheral smear examination

HEME

P 262 A 36-year-old woman who takes no medicines has persistent fatigue and weakness. Vital signs are normal. Hemoglobin is 11.4 g/dL and white blood cell count is 4700/microliter. Serum electrolytes are normal. Which of the following serum values is most likely to be diagnostic in the patient?

A. Lactic dehydrogenase 210 units/L
B. Thyroid-stimulating hormone level 4 mU/mL
C. Cholesterol 330 mg/dL
D. Ferritin 8 ng/mL
E. C-reactive protein 4 mg/L

GI/N, HEME

P 263 Which of the following is the pathophysiologic mechanism that results in iron deficiency in the patient who has celiac disease?

A. Gastrointestinal bleeding due to hypocoagulable state
B. Extravascular hemolysis
C. Decreased marrow hematopoiesis
D. Release of phosphate from myeloid cells
E. Decreased gastrointestinal absorption of iron

REPRO, CV

P 264 In the 21st week of gestation, a 33-year-old primigravida has persistent blood pressure levels of 160/102 mm Hg associated with proteinuria. Which of the following is contraindicated?

A. Hydralazine
B. Methyldopa
C. Nifedipine
D. Labetalol
E. Captopril

MS

P 265 A 33-year-old woman has a 2-month history of disturbing drawing and pulling sensations in both lower legs. The discomfort occurs only at rest and is immediately relieved by movement. Which of the following is the most likely etiology?

A. Iron deficiency
B. Muscle glycogen deficiency
C. Heightened creatine kinase activity
D. Estrogen deficiency
E. Hypercortisolism

GU

P 266 A 22-year-old man has a testicular mass. A germ cell testicular tumor is most likely when there is an elevated serum concentration of which of the following?

A. Testosterone
B. Luteinizing hormone
C. Prolactin
D. Alpha-fetoprotein
E. Adrenocorticotrophic hormone

GI/N

P 267 A 56-year-old man has alcoholic cirrhosis. Elevation in the serum concentration of which of the following is most suggestive of the development of hepatocellular carcinoma?

A. Alanine aminotransferase
B. Anti-smooth muscle antibodies
C. Ant-actin antibodies
D. Alpha-fetoprotein
E. Monoclonal M protein

GU

P 268 A 62-year-old man has red-colored urine for 2 days. Urine dipstick is positive for blood. Microscopic examination of the urine sediment shows no red blood cells. Which of the following is the most likely diagnosis?

A. Beeturia
B. Phenazopyridine ingestion
C. Porphyria
D. Intravascular hemolysis
E. Carcinoma of the kidney

DERM

P 269 A 10-year-old girl has a 1-week history of low-grade fever, rhinorrhea, and headache followed by onset of a bilateral erythematous malar rash and circumoral pallor. No other rash is present. Which of the following is the most likely diagnosis?

A. Systemic lupus erythematosus
B. Rubella
C. Erythema infectiosum
D. Herpangina
E. Hypersensitivity vasculitis

ID

P 270 An asymptomatic 29-year-old man with positive HIV serology should be considered to have AIDS when which of the following is met?

A. CD4 lymphocyte count is greater than 400 cells/microliter
B. HIV viral load is <200 copies
C. Serum IgM concentration is <50 mg/dL
D. CD lymphocyte percentage is >20%
E. CD lymphocyte count is <200 cells/microliter

ID

P 271 A 33-year-old woman with AIDS has a CD4 count of 48 cells/microL. Her tuberculin skin test shows 7 mm induration. She is varicella-zoster seronegative. Which of the following is not a recommended prophylactic therapy?

A. Zoster vaccination
B. Trimethoprim-sulfamethoxazole
C. Isoniazid
D. Influenza vaccine
E. Pneumococcal vaccine

NEURO, ENDO

P 272 A 71-year-old woman with diabetes mellitus has numbness and tingling of both feet and lower legs. Which of the following neurologic signs is least likely to be noted upon examination?

A. Impaired proprioception
B. Absent ankle deep tendon reflexes
C. Loss of light touch
D. Loss of vibratory sensation
E. Extensor Babinski response

NEURO, ENDO

P 273 A 47-year-old man has the sudden onset of foot drop due to common peroneal nerve palsy. Which of the following is the most likely underlying condition?

A. Graves' disease
B. Syndrome of inappropriate anti-diuretic hormone
C. Guillain-Barré syndrome
D. Diabetes mellitus
E. Myasthenia gravis

GI/N, NEURO, ENDO

P 274 A 60-year-old man who has type 1 diabetes mellitus has autonomic neuropathy involving the gastrointestinal tract. Which of the following is the most likely manifestation?

A. Water brash
B. Hematochezia
C. Malabsorption syndrome
D. Small bowel obstruction
E. Nocturnal diarrhea

CV, ENDO

P 275 Clinical testing in a 67-year-old man with diabetes mellitus demonstrates a lack in variation of heart rate during deep breathing and Valsalva maneuvers. The patient is at increased risk for which of the following?

A. Unstable angina pectoris
B. Diastolic heart failure
C. 3rd degree atrioventricular block
D. Sudden cardiac death
E. Respiratory acidosis

CV, NEURO, ENDO

P 276 A 67-year-old diabetic man has lightheadedness when arising from bed. While sitting, blood pressure is 116/78 mm Hg with a pulse of 80/min. Standing blood pressure is 90/62 mm Hg with a pulse of 81/min. Which of the following is the most likely pathophysiologic mechanism causing the observed hemodynamic response?

A. Autonomic insufficiency
B. Hypovolemia
C. Parasympathetic nervous system dysfunction
D. Deficiency of gamma amino butyric acid receptors
E. Extrapyramidal nervous system dysfunction

REPRO

P 277 Presence of which of the following differentiates the typical presentation of abruptio placentae from placenta previa?

A. Passage of blood clots
B. 1st trimester bleeding
C. Serum anti-phospholipid antibodies
D. Uterine contractions
E. Thrombocytosis

REPRO

P 278 A 29-year-old woman has had three spontaneous pregnancy losses in a row. Each pregnancy ended in the 11th to 13th week of gestation. Which of the following is the most likely underlying maternal condition?

A. Reactive hypoglycemia
B. Presence of anti-thyroid peroxidase antibodies
C. Presence of anti-parietal cell antibodies
D. Membranous ventricular septal defect
E. Presence of anti-phospholipid antibodies

ID, HEME

P 279 A 14-year-old boy with sickle cell anemia has had repeated infarctions of his spleen. Which of the following is appropriate therapy?

A. Daily oral penicillin
B. Monthly intramuscular streptomycin
C. Annual herpes zoster vaccination
D. Annual parenteral pegfilgrastim (Neulasta)
E. Monthly parenteral erythropoietin

NEURO, GI/N

P 280 A 52-year-old man with advanced chronic liver disease has hepatic encephalopathy manifest by confusion. Neurologic examination shows bilateral asterixis. Which of the following is preferred initial therapy?

A. Administration of oral spironolactone
B. Administration of Kayexalate enema
C. Administration of oral clindamycin
D. Ingestion of diet containing 125 g protein daily
E. Administration of lactulose enema

GU, GI/N

P 281 A 56-year-old woman has severe chronic liver disease due to alcohol abuse. Which of the following conditions is most likely to precipitate hepatic encephalopathy?

A. Ingestion of low-protein diet
B. Inhalation of 40% oxygen
C. Intake of zinc-containing antacids
D. Hypokalemia
E. Development of ascites

GU

P 282 Upon completing a marathon run, a 29-year-old man has nausea, vomiting, and is in a confused state. Serum sodium is 119 mEq/L. Which of the following is the most likely cause of the hyponatremia?

A. Inadequate renal reabsorption of sodium
B. Low sodium concentration in sweat
C. Ingestion of excess water during race
D. Ingestion of a nonsteroidal anti-inflammatory before the race
E. Ingestion of a high-protein diet before the race

NEURO

P 283 Presence of which of the following differentiates a seizure from a transient ischemic attack?

A. Numbness
B. Diplopia
C. Weakness
D. Headache
E. Visual hallucinations

ENDO, NEURO

P 284 A 46-year-old man has a subarachnoid hemorrhage due to rupture of a cerebral aneurysm. Ten hours later his urinary volume increases to 425 mL/hr. Serum sodium is 156 mEq/L. Which of the following is the most likely complication of the hemorrhage?

A. Diabetes insipidus
B. Hyperglycemic, nonketotic state
C. Hyperhidrosis
D. Syndrome of inappropriate anti-diuretic hormone secretion
E. Acute adrenal insufficiency

ENDO, NEURO

P 285 A 16-year-old man has generalized seizures for which he is transported to the emergency department. Lorazepam, phenytoin, and phenobarbital do not end the seizure activity. Which of the following is the most likely diagnosis?

A. Epilepsy
B. Arteriovenous malformation in the brain
C. Multiple sclerosis
D. Hypoglycemia
E. Hypercalcemia

GI/N

P 286 Which of the following is considered to be the pathophysiologic mechanism causing symptoms in dumping syndrome?

A. Postprandial hypoglycemia
B. Shift of fluid from circulation into bowel
C. Heightened vagal tone
D. Excess secretion of serotonin
E. Decreased adrenal secretion of catecholamines

ID, DERM, GU

P 287 A 32-year-old woman has asymptomatic lesions on her vulva. Examination shows condyloma acuminate. Infection due to which of the following is most likely?

A. Herpes simplex virus
B. Coxsackievirus
C. *Haemophilus ducreyi*
D. *Donovania granulomatis*
E. Human papillomavirus

PSY/LE, NEURO

P 288 Presence of which of the following differentiates delirium tremens from alcoholic hallucinosis?

A. Somnolence
B. Auditory hallucinations
C. Hypotension
D. Disorientation
E. Alcohol abstinence before onset

PSY/LE, GI/N

P 289 A 57-year-old man with a long history of chronic alcohol abuse has the acute onset of delirium tremens. In addition to benzodiazepine therapy, which of the following should be administered?

A. Vitamin B_{12}
B. Folinic acid
C. Bromocriptine
D. Paraldehyde
E. Thiamine

GI/N

P 290 A 3-week-old male infant has postprandial vomiting. Hypertrophic pyloric stenosis is diagnosed. Neonatal ingestion of which of the following is most likely associated with this diagnosis?

A. Nonaspirin, nonselective nonsteroidal anti-inflammatory
B. Medium-chain fatty acid formula
C. Increased dietary proportion of whey to casein
D. Cephalosporin
E. Macrolide

ENDO

P 291 Which of the following classes of hypoglycemic medicines reduces gastrointestinal absorption of carbohydrate?

A. Insulin
B. Sulfonylureas
C. Thiazolidines
D. Alpha-glucosidase inhibitors
E. Meglitinides

ENDO

P 292 Which of the following is the mechanism of action of thiazolidinediones in therapy of type 2 diabetes mellitus?

A. Suppress hepatic glucose production
B. Reduce gastrointestinal absorption of carbohydrate
C. Increase sensitivity to insulin
D. Increase pancreatic secretion of insulin
E. Inhibit autoimmune destruction of pancreas

PUL

P 293 A 27-year-old man with asthma has increased dyspnea and wheezing 1 hour after having been a passenger on a 4-hour commercial airline flight. Which of the following environmental factors in the aircraft cabin is the most likely cause of the respiratory symptoms?

A. Reduced cabin pressure
B. Reduced oxygen pressure
C. Low humidity
D. Transmission of airborne pathogens
E. Vibration of aircraft

EENT, DERM, ID

P 294 A 7-year-old boy has a 5-day history of fever and photophobia. Examination shows conjunctivitis, "strawberry" tongue, and cracked, red lips. A diagnosis of Kawasaki disease is made. Which of the following is the preferred initial therapy?

A. Intravenous methylprednisolone
B. Intravenous immune globulin plus aspirin
C. Intravenous cyclophosphamide
D. Oral aspirin alone
E. Intravenous rituximab (Rituxan)

CV

P 295 Which of the following is the major complication of untreated Kawasaki disease?

A. Autoimmune hemolytic anemia
B. Cholestatic hepatitis
C. Necrotizing pneumonia
D. Coronary artery aneurysm
E. Renal papillary necrosis

REPRO

P 296 A 36-year-old woman who has hyperlipidemia and who smokes cigarettes seeks counseling concerning oral contraceptive therapy. Her aunt and mother both died of ovarian cancer. Which of the following is appropriate counseling for the patient concerning the oral contraceptives?

A. Decrease risk of coronary heart disease
B. Decrease risk of ovarian cancer
C. Oral contraceptive therapy is appropriate for the patient
D. Lower serum triglycerides
E. Lower blood pressure

REPRO, GU

P 297 A 34-year-old woman has a 7-month history of oligomenorrhea. Examination shows an obese, hirsute woman. Which of the following serum laboratory values would be consistent with a diagnosis of polycystic ovary syndrome?

A. Increased luteinizing hormone
B. Decreased testosterone
C. Decreased estrogen
D. Decreased insulin
E. Increased serotonin

ENDO

P 298 A 61-year-old woman has a 4-month history of enlarging hands and feet. A diagnosis of acromegaly is made. In addition to increased secretion of growth hormone, there is increased secretion of which of the following?

A. Thyroid-stimulating hormone
B. Corticotrophin
C. Follicle-stimulating hormone
D. Vasopressin
E. Prolactin

CV

P 299 A 40-year-old woman has a 3-month history of paroxysmal episodes of diffuse headache, sweating, palpitations, and anxiety. Each episode lasts approximately 30 minutes. Examination shows sitting blood pressure 200/120 mm Hg with pulse rate 100/min. Standing blood pressure is 170/106 mm Hg with pulse rate of 114/min. Which of the following is the most appropriate laboratory test?

A. 24-hour urine assay for cortisol
B. 24-hour urine assay for catecholamines
C. 24-hour urine assay for sodium and potassium
D. Plasma renin activity
E. 2-hour glucose tolerance test

GU, PSY/LE

P 300 A 56-year-old man takes sildenafil for therapy of erectile dysfunction. He now has new-onset hypertension. Addition of which of the following medicines is considered to have the greatest risk of causing profound hypotension?

　A. Hydrochlorothiazide
　B. Captopril
　C. Verapamil
　D. Doxazosin
　E. Propranolol

MS, GU

P 301 A 72-year-old man with type 2 diabetes mellitus and coronary heart disease has a blood urea nitrogen value of 38 mg/dL and a serum creatinine concentration of 1.9 mg/dL. Which of the following is the most appropriate advice for the patient?

　A. Avoid nonaspirin, nonselective, nonsteroidal anti-inflammatory agents
　B. Avoid thiazide diuretics
　C. Limit daily fluid intake to 1000 cc
　D. Avoid aspirin
　E. Isometric exercise is preferable to rhythmic exercise

GU, CV

P 302 A 59-year-old woman has hypertension for which she takes lisinopril therapy. The patient now has painful osteoarthritis for which ibuprofen is prescribed. Which of the following is the most appropriate intervention to be taken in 10 to 14 days?

　A. Check blood urea nitrogen/serum creatinine ratio
　B. Check serum potassium concentration
　C. Obtain complete blood count
　D. Check fasting blood sugar level
　E. Check urine for proteinuria

NEURO, EENT

P 303 Presence of which of the following differentiates positional vertigo from presyncope related to orthostatic hypotension?

　A. Symptoms occur when arising from bed
　B. Unstable gait
　C. Vertigo occurs when bending head back to look up
　D. Vertigo is associated with pallor
　E. Vertigo is associated with dimmed vision

HEME

P 304 An 18-year-old man has a severe frontal headache after exposure to a poorly ventilated fuel-burning stove. A diagnosis of carbon monoxide poisoning is made. Which of the following is the preferred therapy?

A. High-flow inhalation of oxygen via face mask
B. Administration of intravenous methylene blue
C. Administration of intravenous sodium bicarbonate
D. Positive end-expiratory pressure breathing treatment
E. Administration of oral N-acetylcysteine

ID, GU

P 305 A 33-year-old healthy, nonpregnant woman has a 3-day history of vaginal burning and dysuria. A vaginal discharge then is noted. Presence of which of the following is most suggestive of *Trichomonas vaginitis*?

A. Clue cells on wet mount preparation
B. Pyuria
C. Inguinal adenopathy
D. Gram-negative cocci in vaginal specimen
E. Strawberry cervix on physical examination

ID, GU

P 306 A 29-year-old healthy, nonpregnant woman has a vaginal discharge. A diagnosis of bacterial vaginosis is made based upon the presence of clue cells. Which of the following best describes clue cells?

A. Macrophages containing gram-positive cocci
B. Atypical monocytes
C. Polymorphonuclear cells with inclusion bodies
D. Vaginal epithelium cells with adherent bacteria
E. Macrophages containing azure bodies

ID, GU

P 307 A 29-year-old healthy, nonpregnant woman has gonococcal urethritis. Which of the following is the preferred therapy?

A. Ceftriaxone plus doxycycline
B. Nafcillin
C. Ciprofloxacin
D. Ceftriaxone alone
E. Ceftriaxone plus trimethoprim-sulfamethoxazole

ID, GU

P 308 A 35-year-old man has a 2-day history of fever, urinary frequency, and perineal pain. Examination shows a very tender, swollen prostate. Urinalysis shows 25 leukocytes/high-power field. Culture of the urine indicates infection by *Escherichia coli*. Which of the following is the preferred oral regimen of therapy?

   A. Ciprofloxacin for 5 weeks
   B. Ampicillin for 10 days
   C. Levofloxacin for 10 days
   D. Cephalexin for 10 days
   E. Cefaclor for 5 weeks

ID, GU

P 309 A 41-year-old man has acute bacterial prostatitis manifest by fever, dysuria, and urinary frequency. Which of the following is the most likely infecting organism?

   A. *Yersinia*
   B. *Neisseria*
   C. *Gardnerella*
   D. *Bacteroides*
   E. *Pseudomonas*

HEME, CV

P 310 A 74-year-old woman has acute dyspnea and hemoptysis. In the past 2 months she has lost 8 pounds and has a poor appetite. Blood pressure is 112/72 mm Hg, pulse is 112/min, and respiratory rate is 23/min. Examination shows a thin, noncyanotic patient. Lungs are clear to auscultation. Examination of the heart and abdomen is normal. Which of the following is the most likely underlying diagnosis?

   A. Systemic lupus erythematosus
   B. Factor V Leiden mutation
   C. Mural thrombus of the left ventricle
   D. Adenocarcinoma of the pancreas
   E. Idiopathic thrombocytopenic purpura

Section Two 2

Answers to Performance Questions

The ⟳ symbol represents links to related questions and key information in the Essentials section.

P 001   (A) Digoxin
            ⟳   Answer E 013

P 002   (A) Oral administration of B-complex vitamins
            ⟳   Answer E 002

P 003   (B) Oral verapamil
            ⟳   Answer E 001

P 004   (C) Normal pressure hydrocephalus
            ⟳   Answer E 003

P 005   (D) Glucose-6 phosphate dehydrogenase deficiency
            ⟳   Answer E 006

P 006   (D) Thyroid-stimulating hormone 22 microU/mL
            ⟳   Answer E 003

P 007   (C) Diastolic heart failure
            ⟳   Answers E 001

P 008   (C) Anginal equivalent
            ⟳   Answers E 001 and E 007

P 009   (D) Hypertrophic obstructive cardiomyopathy
            ⟳   Answers E 001 and E 007

P 010 (A) Niacin
 ↩ Answer E 008

P 011 (B) Verapamil
 ↩ Answer E 009

P 012 (C) Intravenous administration of octreotide
 ↩ Answer E 012

P 013 (A) Adverse effect of verapamil
 ↩ Answer E 013

P 014 (B) Non-Hodgkin's lymphoma
 ↩ Answer E 014

P 015 (D) Constrictive pericarditis
 ↩ Answer E 014

P 016 (A) Transesophageal echocardiogram
 ↩ Answer E 015

P 017 (A) Acute cholecystitis
 ↩ Answer E 010

P 018 (B) Primary biliary cirrhosis
 ↩ Answer E 016

P 019 (B) Initiate angiotensin-converting enzyme inhibitor therapy
 ↩ Answer E 017

P 020 (C) Systemic lupus erythematosus
 ↩ Answer E 018

P 021 (C) Autonomic insufficiency
 ↩ Answer E 019

P 022 (D) Stand or sit upright for 30 minutes after taking medication
 ↩ Answer E 020

Section 2 ■ Answers to Performance Questions

P 023 (A) Insulin dosage may increase due to hyperglycemic effect of niacin
⟲ Answer E 008

P 024 (D) Propranolol
⟲ Answer E 021

P 025 (D) Recurrent myocardial infarction
⟲ Answer E 022

P 026 (B) Mitochondria
⟲ Answer E 016

P 027 (B) Alpha-fetoprotein
⟲ Answer E 012

P 028 (C) White blood cell count 2100/microL
⟲ Answer E 018

P 029 (D) Pheochromocytoma
⟲ Answer E 019

P 030 (D) Cosyntropin stimulation test
⟲ Answer E 019

P 031 (E) Serum creatine kinase and troponin levels
⟲ Answer E 024

P 032 (C) Right heart failure
⟲ Answer E 025

P 033 (B) Obtain thyroid function values every 3 to 4 months
⟲ Answer E 026

P 034 (C) Amaurosis fugax
⟲ Answer E 027

P 035 (B) Tourette's syndrome
⟲ Answer E 028

P 036   (E) Oats
        ↩ Answer E 029

P 037   (B) Heightened vagal tone
        ↩ Answer E 023

P 038   (D) Pulmonary hypertension
        ↩ Answer E 025

P 039   (D) Anorectal manometry
        ↩ Answer E 030

P 040   (D) Cataracts
        ↩ Answer E 031

P 041   (B) Avoid pregnancy while taking lithium
        ↩ Answer E 026

P 042   (A) Adenocarcinoma of the stomach
        ↩ Answer E 032

P 043   (B) Hypokalemia
        ↩ Answer E 033

P 044   (A) Aseptic meningitis
        ↩ Answer E 035

P 045   (C) Corneal ulceration
        ↩ Answer E 036

P 046   (E) Scleroderma
        ↩ Answer E 044

P 047   (A) ELISA test
        ↩ Answer E 037

P 048   (C) Oral allopurinol
        ↩ Answer E 038

Section 2 ■ Answers to Performance Questions

P 049   (B) Elevated angiotensin-converting enzyme
        Answer E 039

P 050   (C) Avoid extended wear of the soft lens
        Answer E 036

P 051   (B) Diabetes mellitus
        Answer E 040

P 052   (D) Acute dissection of the thoracic aorta
        Answer E 042

P 053   (C) Perform duplex carotid artery ultrasound
        Answer E 027

P 054   (C) Initiate therapy with a bisphosphonate
        Answer E 031

P 055   (B) Hypokalemia
        Answer E 033

P 056   (C) Administration of intravenous glucose and insulin
        Answer E 034

P 057   (D) Scleroderma
        Answer E 044

P 058   (A) pH 7.48, PaO_2 66 mm Hg, $PaCO_2$ 28 mm Hg
        Answer E 039

P 059   (C) Decreased carbon monoxide diffusing capacity
        Answer E 039

P 060   (B) Hypersegmented neutrophiles
        Answer E 051

P 061   (E) Henoch-Schönlein purpura
        Answer E 049

P 062 (C) Methylmalonic acid
↩ Answer E 051

P 063 (C) Transesophageal echocardiography
↩ Answer E 042

P 064 (B) Do not take medication with antacids
↩ Answer E 043

P 065 (B) Metoprolol
↩ Answer E 042

P 066 (B) Abnormal position sense
↩ Answer E 051

P 067 (C) Receive monthly vitamin B_{12} injections
↩ Answer E 051

P 068 (C) Lack of intrinsic factor production
↩ Answer E 051

P 069 (B) Crohn's disease
↩ Answer E 058

P 070 (A) Decreased arterial compliance
↩ Answer E 059

P 071 (C) Initiate thiazide therapy
↩ Answer E 059

P 072 (C) Romberg test
↩ Answer E 060

P 073 (C) Hyperthyroidism
↩ Answer E 059

P 074 (B) Autonomic insufficiency
↩ Answer E 054

Section 2 ■ **Answers to Performance Questions**

P 075   (D) Hypovolemia
          ↩ Answer E 054

P 076   (C) Diabetes mellitus
          ↩ Answer E 054

P 077   (C) Ventricular wall stretching
          ↩ Answer E 069

P 078   (D) Normal plasma Nt-BNP
          ↩ Answer E 069

P 079   (E) Small cell carcinoma of lung
          ↩ Answer E 057

P 080   (E) *Pseudomonas aeruginosa*
          ↩ Answer E 056

P 081   (B) Platelet count
          ↩ Answer E 055

P 082   (D) Bronchiectasis
          ↩ Answer E 056

P 083   (E) Hydrochlorothiazide
          ↩ Answer E 026

P 084   (B) Avoid pregnancy
          ↩ Answer E 026

P 085   (A) Unilateral character of visual symptoms
          ↩ Answer E 027

P 086   (A) Prednisone
          ↩ Answer E 031

P 087   (E) Gastric adenocarcinoma
          ↩ Answer E 032

P 088 (B) Tissue insulin resistance
       ↩ Answer E 032

P 089 (B) Erythema migrans
       ↩ Answer E 037

P 090 (D) Oral allopurinol
       ↩ Answer E 038

P 091 (D) Normal FEV 1 sec/FVC ratio
       ↩ Answer E 039

P 092 (B) Hyperuricemic nephropathy
       ↩ Answer E 038

P 093 (C) Metoprolol
       ↩ Answer E 045

P 094 (B) Decrease ventricular preload
       ↩ Answer E 046

P 095 (A) Hypomagnesemia
       ↩ Answer E 047

P 096 (A) Ability to wrinkle forehead on affected side
       ↩ Answer E 037

P 097 (C) Long QT interval syndrome
       ↩ Answer E 064

P 098 (D) Verapamil
       ↩ Answer E 048

P 099 (E) Hypertension
       ↩ Answer E 049

P 100 (D) Red blood cell casts
       ↩ Answer E 049

Section 2 ▪ Answers to Performance Questions

P 101   (B) Pernicious anemia
            ↩ Answer E 050

P 102   (C) Pernicious anemia
            ↩ Answer E 051

P 103   (A) Macrocytosis
            ↩ Answer E 050

P 104   (A) Elevated plasma adrenocorticotropin level
            ↩ Answer E 065

P105   (B) Adrenal insufficiency
            ↩ Answer E 065

P 106   (C) White blood cell count 2000/microL
            ↩ Answers E 018, E 052

P 107   (B) Avoid direct sunlight
            ↩ Answer E 052

P 108   (E) Serum anti-nuclear antibody titer
            ↩ Answer E 052

P 109   (B) Intranasal beclomethasone
            ↩ Answer E 053

P 110   (B) Coarctation of the aorta
            ↩ Answers E 057, E 170

P 111   (D) No need for endocarditis prophylaxis
            ↩ Answer E 079

P 112   (E) Verapamil
            ↩ Answer E 007

P 113   (B) Thallium stress cardiac testing
            ↩ Answer E 001

P 114 (A) Non-Hodgkin's lymphoma
↩ Answer E 014

P 115 (D) Move chin from side to side
↩ Answer E 037

P 116 (B) Paget's disease of bone
↩ Answer E 066

P 117 (B) Significant aortic stenosis is likely to occur in adulthood
↩ Answer E 057

P 118 (D) Verapamil
↩ Answer E 013

P 119 (A) Diltiazem
↩ Answer E 013

P 120 (B) Elevated urinary hydroxyproline
↩ Answer E 066

P 121 (A) Dilated cardiomyopathy
↩ Answer E 013

P 122 (C) Nadolol
↩ Answer E 012

P 123 (D) Alpha-fetoprotein
↩ Answer E 012

P 124 (B) ST segment elevation
↩ Answer E 007

P 125 (A) Do not become pregnant while on therapy
↩ Answer E 070

P 126 (B) Pitting of nails
↩ Answer E 082

Section 2 ■ **Answers to Performance Questions**

P 127 (B) Panic disorder
↩ Answer E 093

P 128 (E) Withdraw medication over 1 week if it is to be discontinued
↩ Answer E 070

P 129 (D) "Sharpened pencil" appearance of fingers
↩ Answer E 082

P 130 (A) Angiotensin-converting enzyme inhibitor
↩ Answer E 070

P 131 (C) Captopril
↩ Answer E 070

P 132 (A) Betamethasone with clotrimazole (Lotrisone)
↩ Answer E 081

P 133 (A) Hydrochlorothiazide
↩ Answer E 070

P 134 (D) Hydrochlorothiazide
↩ Answer E 070

P 135 (D) Thiazide
↩ Answer E 070

P 136 (B) Glucagon
↩ Answer E 085

P 137 (D) Potassium hydroxide preparation of scales
↩ Answer E 081

P 138 (A) Selective serotonin receptor inhibitors
↩ Answer E 071

P 139 (E) Phosphodiesterase 5 inhibitors
↩ Answer E 071

P 140 (B) Place clothes worn before diagnosis in plastic bag for 10 days
↩ Answer E 072

P 141 (E) *Streptococcus*
↩ Answer E 080

P 142 (C) Lichen planus
↩ Answer E 072

P 143 (C) Metronidazole gel
↩ Answer E 072

P 144 (E) Saliva may remain contagious for 6 months
↩ Answer E 080

P 145 (B) Alcohol ingestion
↩ Answer E 072

P 146 (B) Cor pulmonale
↩ Answer E 073

P 147 (C) Verapamil
↩ Answers E 013 and E 087

P 148 (B) Pa_{O_2} 60 mm Hg, Pa_{CO_2} 60 mm Hg
↩ Answer E 073

P 149 (E) Mitral valve prolapse
↩ Answer E 079

P 150 (D) St. John's wort
↩ Answer E 074

P 151 (C) Haloperidol
↩ Answer E 074

P 152 (D) Chronic obstructive lung disease
↩ Answer E 087

Section 2 ■ **Answers to Performance Questions**

P 153 (D) Infusion of 0.9% saline
↩ Answer E 091

P 154 (B) Serotonin syndrome
↩ Answer E 074

P 155 (E) Autoimmune destruction of pancreatic B cells
↩ Answer E 085

P 156 (B) Check blood pressure in 10 to 14 days
↩ Answers E 016, E 075

P 157 (E) Indomethacin
↩ Answer E 075

P 158 (A) Have liver function tests performed every 4 to 8 weeks
↩ Answer E 076

P 159 (A) Do not take acetaminophen in dosage > 2.0 g/day
↩ Answer E 077

P 160 (A) Mechanical heart valve in aortic position
↩ Answer E 079

P 161 (A) Level of 24-hour urinary excretion of uric acid
↩ Answer E 078

P 162 (E) Avoid ingestion of alcohol
↩ Answer E 078

P 163 (D) Reduce ingestion of red meat and shellfish
↩ Answer E 078

P 164 (B) Leg claudication
↩ Answer E 087

P 165 (D) Elevated serum luteinizing hormone
↩ Answer E 086

P 166 (D) Waist-to-hip fat ratio
↩ Answer E 085

P 167 (A) HLA-DR3 gene
↩ Answer E 085

P 168 (D) Stool for occult blood
↩ Answer E 084

P 169 (C) Triglycerides
↩ Answer E 083

P 170 (D) Diverticulosis
↩ Answer E 083

P 171 (C) No antibiotic therapy
↩ Answer E 088

P 172 (D) Orthostatic hypotension
↩ Answer E 092

P 173 (E) Sublingual lorazepam (Ativan)
↩ Answer E 093

P 174 (B) Normal saline
↩ Answer E 091

P 175 (E) Serum D-dimer level of 400 nanogram/mL
↩ Answer E 105

P 176 (E) Avoid pregnancy
↩ Answer E 103

P 177 (C) Serum D-dimer level of 400 ng/mL
↩ Answer E 105

P 178 (D) Captopril
↩ Answer E 103

Section 2 ■ **Answers to Performance Questions**

P 179 (C) Outpatient treatment with clarithromycin
↩ Answer E 102

P 180 (E) *Pseudomonas aeruginosa*
↩ Answer E 102

P 181 (D) Tolerated as well as in nonasthmatic
↩ Answer E 101

P 182 (D) Hotel showers
↩ Answer E 102

P 183 (D) Legionnaires' disease
↩ Answer E 102

P 184 (A) Partially hydrogenated coffee creamer
↩ Answer E 100

P 185 (E) Pneumonia with effusion
↩ Answer E 104

P 186 (A) t-PA
↩ Answer E 097

P 187 (E) Hyponatremia
↩ Answer E 104

P 188 (B) Myocardial infarction
↩ Answer E 096

P 189 (A) Gastroparesis
↩ Answer E 095

P 190 (D) Nephrotic syndrome
↩ Answer E 104

P 191 (E) Intravenous alteplase
↩ Answer E 097

P 192 (B) Nuclear scintigraphy after radioactive-labeled meal
　　　　Answer E 095

P 193 (C) Ofloxacin
　　　　Answer E 099

P 194 (C) Zoster rash may appear in 24 to 48 hours
　　　　Answer E 098

P 195 (D) Serum to ascites albumin gradient
　　　　Answer E 094

P 196 (D) Spontaneous bacterial peritonitis
　　　　Answer E 094

P 197 (D) *Giardia lamblia*
　　　　Answer E 113

P 198 (A) Axillary temperature of 103.6°F
　　　　Answer E 113

P 199 (E) *Cryptosporidium*
　　　　Answer E 113

P 200 (B) Irritable bowel syndrome
　　　　Answer E 113

P 201 (D) Nafcillin
　　　　Answer E 106

P 202 (E) Arteriovenous fistula
　　　　Answer E 107

P 203 (A) Healthy 22-year-old nurse
　　　　Answer E 110

P 204 (E) Sore throat
　　　　Answer E 111

Section 2 ■ **Answers to Performance Questions**   233

P 205   (D) Hyperthyroidism
↩ Answer E 107

P 206   (A) Nonaspirin, nonselective, nonsteroidal anti-inflammatory
↩ Answer E 114

P 207   (D) Na − (Cl + HCO$_3$)
↩ Answer E 108

P 208   (A) 47-year-old healthy woman
↩ Answer E 110

P 209   (D) Lumbar puncture
↩ Answer E 112

P 210   (D) Epidural blood patch
↩ Answer E 112

P 211   (E) Assurance to patient that symptoms disappear after delivery
↩ Answer E 109

P 212   (D) Hydrocortisone foam enemas
↩ Answer E 114

P 213   (C) Anti–thyroid-stimulating hormone receptor antibodies
↩ Answer E 111

P 214   (B) Production of lactic acid
↩ Answer E 108

P 215   (A) Flexible sigmoidoscopy
↩ Answer E 114

P 216   (D) Serum thyroid-stimulating hormone level
↩ Answer E 109

P 217   (E) Chocolate ice cream
↩ Answer E 115

P 218 (A) Increased anion gap metabolic acidosis
        Answer E 108

P 219 (D) Methimazole
        Answer E 111

P 220 (D) Ranitidine at bedtime
        Answer E 115

P 221 (B) Serum thyroid stimulating hormone level
        Answer E 111

P 222 (B) Colon cancer
        Answer E 114

P 223 (E) Gastroesophageal reflux
        Answer E 115

P 224 (B) Proteinuria
        Answer E 118

P 225 (E) Seizures
        Answer E 118

P 226 (E) Recurrent fetal loss
        Answer E 118

P 227 (C) Endothelial dysfunction
        Answer E 118

P 228 (D) Transvaginal ultrasonography
        Answer E 119

P 229 (C) History of bipolar coagulation sterilization
        Answer E 119

P 230 (D) Immune due to hepatitis B vaccination
        Answer E 120

Section 2 ■ Answers to Performance Questions

P 231 (C) Chlorpromazine (Thorazine)
↩ Answer E 122

P 232 (E) Hemolytic anemia
↩ Answer E 122

P 233 (E) Ascending cholangitis
↩ Answer E 122

P 234 (D) Anti-mitochondrial
↩ Answer E 122

P 235 (B) Ratio of serum AST/ALT is >2:1
↩ Answer E 122

P 236 (B) Ibuprofen
↩ Answer E 123

P 237 (E) Selective serotonin reuptake inhibitor
↩ Answer E 124

P 238 (A) Anion gap of 18 mEq/L
↩ Answer E 127

P 239 (E) Lactic acidosis
↩ Answer E 128

P 240 (A) Heavy alcohol intake
↩ Answer E 128

P 241 (B) Do not take metformin on morning of study
↩ Answer E 128

P 242 (D) Azithromycin
↩ Answer E 129

P 243 (B) Lidocaine
↩ Answer E 130

P 244 (E) Administration of nebulized albuterol
       ↺ Answer E 130

P 245 (D) Flattening of T waves with prominent U waves
       ↺ Answer E 130

P 246 (A) Anti-acetylcholine
       ↺ Answer E 131

P 247 (E) Anti–thyroid-stimulating hormone antibodies
       ↺ Answer E 131

P 248 (E) Oral angiotensin-converting enzyme inhibitor
       ↺ Answer E 132

P 249 (B) Deep vein thrombosis
       ↺ Answer E 132

P 250 (C) Hodgkin's disease
       ↺ Answer E 133

P 251 (D) Normal gait
       ↺ Answer E 134

P 252 (E) Fasciculations
       ↺ Answer E 134

P 253 (D) Subclavian steal syndrome
       ↺ Answer E 136

P 254 (E) Percutaneous luminal angioplasty
       ↺ Answer E 136

P 255 (D) Angiotensin-converting enzyme inhibitor
       ↺ Answer E 132

P 256 (B) Do not smoke during pregnancy
       ↺ Answer E 138

Section 2 ■ Answers to Performance Questions

P 257 (E) Orthostatic hypotension
↪ Answer E 134

P 258 (A) History of deep vein thrombosis
↪ Answer E 139

P 259 (A) Increases tissue sensitivity to insulin
↪ Answer E 141

P 260 (E) Glyburide therapy must be replaced by insulin
↪ Answer E 141

P 261 (A) Hemosiderinuria
↪ Answer E 143

P 262 (D) Ferritin 8 ng/mL
↪ Answer E 143

P 263 (E) Decreased gastrointestinal absorption of iron
↪ Answer E 143

P 264 (E) Captopril
↪ Answer E 142

P 265 (A) Iron deficiency
↪ Answer E 143

P 266 (D) Alpha-fetoprotein
↪ Answer E 144

P 267 (D) Alpha-fetoprotein
↪ Answer E 144

P 268 (D) Intravascular hemolysis
↪ Answer E 145

P 269 (C) Erythema infectiosum
↪ Answer E 146

P 270 (E) CD lymphocyte count is <200 cells/microliter
　　　　　↩ Answer E 147

P 271 (E) Pneumococcal vaccine
　　　　　↩ Answer E 148

P 272 (E) Extensor Babinski response
　　　　　↩ Answer E 149

P 273 (D) Diabetes mellitus
　　　　　↩ Answer E 149

P 274 (E) Nocturnal diarrhea
　　　　　↩ Answer E 150

P 275 (D) Sudden cardiac death
　　　　　↩ Answer E 150

P 276 (A) Autonomic insufficiency
　　　　　↩ Answer E 150

P 277 (D) Uterine contractions
　　　　　↩ Answer E 151

P 278 (E) Presence of anti-phospholipid antibodies
　　　　　↩ Answer E 151

P 279 (A) Daily oral penicillin
　　　　　↩ Answer E 152

P 280 (E) Administration of lactulose enema
　　　　　↩ Answer E 153

P 281 (D) Hypokalemia
　　　　　↩ Answer E 153

P 282 (C) Ingestion of excess water during race
　　　　　↩ Answer E 155

P 283 (E) Visual hallucinations
　　　　　↩ Answer E 156

Section 2 ■ Answers to Performance Questions

P 284   (A) Diabetes insipidus
      ↩ Answer E 157

P 285   (D) Hypoglycemia
      ↩ Answer E 158

P 286   (B) Shift of fluid from circulation into bowel
      ↩ Answer E 158

P 287   (E) Human papillomavirus
      ↩ Answer E 159

P 288   (D) Disorientation
      ↩ Answer E 160

P 289   (E) Thiamine
      ↩ Answer E 160

P 290   (E) Macrolide
      ↩ Answer E 161

P 291   (D) Alpha-glucosidase inhibitors
      ↩ Answer E 162

P 292   (C) Increase sensitivity to insulin
      ↩ Answer E 162

P 293   (C) Low humidity
      ↩ Answer E 163

P 294   (B) Intravenous immune globulin plus aspirin
      ↩ Answer E 164

P 295   (D) Coronary artery aneurysm
      ↩ Answer E 164

P 296   (B) Decrease risk of ovarian cancer
      ↩ Answer E 166

P 297   (A) Increased luteinizing hormone
      ↩ Answer E 167

P 298 (E) Prolactin
 Answer E 167

P 299 (B) 24-hour urine assay for catecholamines
 Answer E 167

P 300 (D) Doxazosin
 Answer E 168

P 301 (A) Avoid nonaspirin, nonselective, nonsteroidal anti-inflammatory agents
 Answer E 168

P 302 (B) Check serum potassium concentration
 Answer E 168

P 303 (C) Vertigo occurs when bending head back to look up
 Answer E 171

P 304 (A) High-flow inhalation of oxygen via face mask
 Answer E 172

P 305 (E) Strawberry cervix on physical examination
 Answer E 175

P 306 (D) Vaginal epithelium cells with adherent bacteria
 Answer E 175

P 307 (A) Ceftriaxone plus doxycycline
 Answers E 099, E 175

P 308 (A) Ciprofloxacin for 5 weeks
 Answer E 176

P 309 (E) *Pseudomonas*
 Answer E 176

P 310 (D) Adenocarcinoma of the pancreas
 Answer E 116

Appendix

How You Can Use the NCCPA Content Blueprint to Improve Your Test Performance

The section in the National Commission on Certification of Physician Assistants (NCCPA) website entitled "Exams: Content Blueprint/Task Areas" deserves critical review. Careful consideration of the blueprint will, I believe, result in improved test performance.

The defined NCCPA Task Areas are Applying Basic Concepts, History Taking and Performing Physical Examinations, Using Laboratory and Diagnostic Studies, Formulating Most Likely Diagnosis, Health Maintenance, Clinical Intervention, and Pharmaceutical Therapeutics.

Note: The book's section entitled "Answers to Essentials Questions" is a rich resource that will help you in all Task Areas. Please study the Answers section because it expands on the information that follows.

Applying Basic Concepts

Understanding principles of physiology and pathophysiology should enable the test candidate to correctly answer many PANCE and PANRE questions.

Remember these basic concepts:

Concept 1: Cardiac Function

A cardinal determinant of ventricular function is preload, which relates to the volume of blood in a ventricle at end-diastole. A dilated left ventricle signifies increased preload. Increased preload and the dilated ventricle, in turn, lead to systolic heart failure (SHF). SHF is characterized by a decreased left ventricular ejection fraction and low cardiac output. Typically, the physical examination shows the apical impulse to be displaced to the left and downward in the chest and a S3 gallop is present. The cardinal symptom of SHF is fatigue/weakness.

In contrast, diastolic heart failure (DHF) is due to a stiff left ventricle (decreased compliance). The stiff ventricle is often related to ventricular hypertrophy from increased afterload, a second physiologic determinant of ventricular function.

Increased afterload is caused by either systemic hypertension or aortic valve stenosis. In order to fill the stiff ventricle during diastole, left atrial pressure must increase in order to propel the blood into the ventricle. This increased atrial pressure is transmitted back to the lungs and the patient's symptom is dyspnea. The physical signs of DHF are an apical lift signifying left ventricular hypertrophy and a S4 gallop.

Note the key difference: SHF = fatigue = dilated left ventricle = increased preload. DHF = dyspnea = stiff (noncompliant) left ventricle = increased afterload

You are now able to answer many questions. What is the primary pathophysiologic abnormality in systolic heart failure/diastolic heart failure? Which of the following physical signs is most likely to be noted in the patient who has systolic/diastolic heart failure? What is the pathophysiologic basis for dyspnea in the patient who has diastolic heart failure? A decreased left ventricular ejection fraction is most likely to be noted in a patient with which of the following signs upon cardiac examination?

Concept 2: Cor Pulmonale

Cor pulmonale is heart disease secondary to lung disease. To answer questions correctly, you must know these points:

a. Pulmonary *parenchymal* disease (pulmonary fibrosis or chronic bronchitis) and pulmonary *vascular* disease are the primary causes of cor pulmonale
b. The basic pathophysiologic mechanism in cor pulmonale is increased pulmonary vascular resistance causing pulmonary hypertension

You can now answer important questions: Which of the following is the basic pathophysiologic mechanism in cor pulmonale? Which of the following diseases is most likely to cause cor pulmonale? Which of the following hemodynamic states is characteristic of cor pulmonale?

Concept 3: Syncope

The basic principle in understanding syncope is that all patients who faint share a common pathophysiology, namely, decreased cerebral perfusion. The decreased cerebral blood flow may, in turn, be due to many causes. Cardiovascular causes of syncope include arrhythmia (bradycardia or tachycardia), obstruction to blood flow (aortic valve stenosis, hypertrophic obstructive cardiomyopathy, pulmonary embolism). Reflex syncope is characteristically due to heightened vagal tone. Orthostatic hypotension causing faint may be due to autonomic insufficiency (a defect in the sympathetic reflex arc) or to hypovolemia. Finally, there are psychogenic causes of fainting as may occur in the hysterical patient.

The history then becomes critically important in helping to differentiate among these multiple causes of decreased cerebral perfusion. Syncope while shaving suggests a hypersensitive carotid sinus (vagal response). Heightened vagal tone, as in the anxious patient who is undergoing venipuncture, causes the common faint. Heightened vagal tone, namely, increased parasympathetic activity, is characterized by hypotension and bradycardia. Fainting during an argument or during physical exertion in an older patient raises the possibility of arrhythmia due to myocardial ischemia. In contrast, fainting during argument or exertion in a child or young adult suggests either long QT interval (on electrocardiography) or hypertrophic obstructive cardiomyopathy. Fainting when urinating or defecating is situational syncope related to vagal tone. Finally, syncope when arising from bed indicates orthostatic hypotension. Orthostatic hypotension may be caused by either autonomic insufficiency or hypovolemia. In autonomic insufficiency, the pulse rate does not increase when the standing blood pressure has dropped. In contrast, in hypovolemia, the standing pulse rate is considerably faster than the rate while the patient is recumbent. Here is a typical clinical example: An 81-year-old woman faints when arising from bed. Recumbent blood pressure is 120/70 mm Hg with a pulse of 62/min. Standing blood pressure is 80/58 mm Hg with a pulse of 63/min. In this case, orthostatic hypotension is due to an impaired sympathetic nervous system (autonomic insufficiency) that is commonly noted in the patient who has diabetes mellitus. In contrast, if the fall in blood pressure in this same patient was associated with an increase in pulse rate, for example, from 62 to 88/min, then the cause is hypovolemia as occurs in adrenal insufficiency or hypovolemia due to excessive diuresis.

You are now able to answer many questions. What is the pathophysiologic basis of all patients who faint? What are the typical physical signs during vagal fainting? Which of the following is the most likely cause of syncope in a 14-year-old athlete who faints during a basketball game and in whom physical exam shows an apical lift and double carotid arterial upstroke (bisferiens pulse)? Presence of which of the following differentiates syncope due to autonomic insufficiency from syncope due to hypovolemia? Which of the following activities is most likely to provoke syncope due to carotid sinus hypersensitivity?

Concept 4: Transient Neurologic Symptoms

Transient neurologic symptoms (in most cases, minutes) may be due to transient ischemic attack (TIA), migraine, or seizures. You must understand the difference between "positive" symptoms and "negative" symptoms. Positive symptoms may involve sensory or motor nerves and indicate that the nerve is irritated. Examples of positive symptoms include tingling, burning, jerking, and visual hallucinations. Negative symptoms indicate loss of nerve function. Examples of negative neurologic symptoms include numbness, weakness, or loss of vision.

Transient ischemic attacks always cause *negative* symptoms. In contrast, migraine and seizure activity frequently are associated with *positive* symptoms such as bright lights in the visual fields, jerking, or tingling. Another very important clinical point: in transient ischemic attacks, the symptoms occur at the same time, whereas in migraine or some seizures, the symptoms progress over time. For example, a patient with a TIA has loss of vision and weakness starting at the same time. In contrast, the patient with migraine typically has visual scintillations that slowly progress over the visual fields, or the patient has tingling that starts in one finger and then slowly progresses to involve the hand and arm.

You are now able to answer important questions. Which of the following differentiates a transient ischemic attack from migraine? Negative/positive neurologic symptoms are characteristic of which of the following conditions?

Concept 5: Hypoxemia

Hypoxemia is decreased oxygen in the systemic circulation. Some important mechanisms that cause hypoxemia include hypoventilation, ventilation-perfusion mismatch, and diffusion impairment.

Hypoventilation always causes an increase in P_{CO_2} in the systemic circulation. In room air, hypoventilation is associated with hypoxemia. Clinical examples of hypoventilation include respiratory depression from drug overdose, or brain lesions involving the respiratory center.

Ventilation-perfusion mismatch relates to the balance between lung ventilation and perfusion. Clinical examples of hypoxemia due to this imbalance include obstructive pulmonary disease, pulmonary fibrosis, and chronic pulmonary emboli.

Diffusion impairment results in hypoxemia because there is inefficient transfer of oxygen from alveoli to capillaries. Pulmonary fibrosis is the classic disease characterized by diffusion impairment. Pulmonary fibrosis is considered restrictive lung disease in contrast to chronic bronchitis and emphysema, which are obstructive lung diseases.

How, then, does one differentiate between obstructive and restrictive lung disease? Obstructive lung disease is characterized by increased airway resistance. Restrictive lung disease is characterized by decreased pulmonary compliance. Therefore, a basic lung function test that differentiates between restrictive and obstructive is forced expiratory volume 1 sec/forced vital capacity (FEV 1sec/FVC). In restrictive disease, the ratio is increased and in obstructive lung disease, the ratio is decreased.

You are now able to answer important questions. Which of the following is the pathophysiologic abnormality in restrictive/obstructive lung disease? Which of the following diagnostic tests is preferred to differentiate between restrictive and obstructive lung disease? A patient who has respiratory depression secondary to heroin overdose will have which of the following systemic arterial blood gas values?

Concept 6: Genetic transmission

You should know the inheritance patterns of important disorders. This table will help you answer questions.

Disorder	Genetic Inheritance
Marfan's syndrome	Autosomal dominant
Polycystic kidney	Autosomal dominant
Hypertrophic cardiomyopathy	Autosomal dominant; also sporadic cases

HISTORY TAKING AND PERFORMING PHYSICAL EXAMINATIONS

The History in Differential Diagnosis

You are now aware that the history obtained from the patient can differentiate between TIA and migraine. The activity during which syncope occurs (e.g., arising from bed or during exercise) is extremely important in determining the cause of loss of consciousness.

A thoughtful history can differentiate between angina pectoris and chest pain of noncardiac origin. Angina is a discomfort, not a sharp pain, that lasts continuously for at least 1 minute. Noncardiac pain is often jabbing and momentary, not continuous. Angina pectoris is not associated with chest wall tenderness and is not affected by body position, swallowing, or respiration. In contrast, pericardial pain may be influenced by body position, swallowing, and respiratory movement.

The history is important in differentiating among the many causes of peripheral edema. Edema affecting only one extremity suggests venous or lymphatic obstruction. Bilateral peripheral edema in the patient who suffers from chronic alcohol abuse suggests cirrhosis, portal hypertension, and hypoalbuminemia. Bilateral peripheral edema in the patient with long-standing valvular disease or atherosclerotic heart disease suggests right heart failure. A past history of chest irradiation in a patient presenting with peripheral edema, suggests constrictive pericarditis. The focused physical exam now becomes important. A normal central (jugular) venous pressure (CVP) in the edematous patient suggests liver disease or nephrotic syndrome. However, increased CVP in the edematous patient points toward a diagnosis of right heart failure or constrictive pericarditis.

Here is an important question that tests your physical examination skills. Presence of which of the following differentiates between folate deficiency anemia and vitamin B_{12} deficiency anemia? Answer: normal vibratory sensation and proprioception.

Risk Factors in Disease

The clinician is expected to know risk factors for common diseases. The following table will be helpful to you.

Disorder	Important Risk Factors
Atherosclerotic diseases	Sex, age, family history, dyslipidemia, hypertension, diabetes mellitus, smoking, sedentary lifestyle
Aorta dissection	Hypertension; Marfan's syndrome

Inspection as Part of the Physical Exam

An appropriate exam question would determine your ability to link a physical examination sign upon inspection to a clinical disorder. Here are examples:

Sign Upon Inspection	Significance
Clubbing	Primary or metastatic lung cancer
	Cyanotic congenital heart disease
	Bronchiectasis, pulmonary fibrosis, or lung abscess
	Crohn's disease
	Not a sign of COPD
Jaundice	Hemolysis or obstructive liver disease
Petechiae	Thrombocytopenia
	Vasculitis
	Meningococcemia

(continued)

(continued)

Sign Upon Inspection	Significance
Spider angiomata, palmar erythema	Advanced chronic liver disease
Malar rash in an adult female	Systemic lupus erythematosus
Pitting of nails	Psoriasis
Elevated central venous pressure	Right heart failure
	Constrictive pericarditis
	Pericardial tamponade
	Superior vena cava syndrome
Pallor, periorbital edema	Hypothyroidism
Round face; abdominal striae	Cushing's disease

USING LABORATORY AND DIAGNOSTIC STUDIES

Complete Blood Count

The basic white blood cell count in the blood can be helpful in determining the diagnosis. Acute pericarditis in the patient with systemic lupus erythematosus is associated with leukopenia (often 2500 to 3500/microL), whereas pericarditis due to bacterial infection (purulent pericarditis) typically is characterized by marked leukocytosis.(20,000 to 30,000/microL).

In a question that clearly relates to a patient who has a hematologic disorder, carefully look for the red blood cell volume. Microcytosis suggests iron deficiency anemia or thalassemia. Macrocytosis, importantly, may occur with or without a megaloblastic bone marrow. Megaloblastic anemia with macrocytosis is due to either folate or vitamin B_{12} deficiency. Macrocytosis without megaloblasts is due to hypothyroidism, alcohol intake, or liver disease.

Serum Potassium

a. Hyperkalemia—immediately think of the following causes: renal failure (acute or chronic) and medicines (angiotensin-converting enzyme inhibitors [ACEI], spironolactone, and triamterene)
b. Hypokalemia—immediately think of the following causes: loop-diuretic therapy; diarrhea; tube drainage; and vomiting

You can now answer many questions: Lisinopril therapy is initiated in a 65-year-old man. Which of the following laboratory tests should be performed in 10 days? Which of the following laboratory abnormalities is most likely to be noted in a 44-year-old man with recurrent severe vomiting?

Autoimmune Diseases and Their Antibodies

Laboratory studies provide an important clue between pernicious anemia (PA) and other causes of vitamin B_{12} deficiency anemia. Only pernicious anemia is an autoimmune disorder. Therefore, only in pernicious anemia does the patient's serum have antibodies to intrinsic factor and gastric parietal cells.

Similarly, there are several diseases that cause hyperthyroidism. Only Graves' disease is autoimmune and is associated with extrathyroidal signs (e.g., pretibial myxedema). Solitary toxic thyroid nodule, toxic multinodular goiter, and exogenous hyperthyroidism are not autoimmune and, therefore, are not associated with autoantibody formation.

You should expect that the PANCE and PANRE examinations will have many questions related to autoimmune diseases. The following table should be helpful to you.

Disease	Clinical Character	Antibodies
Systemic lupus	Arthritis, pericarditis, malar rash	Anti-nuclear, anti-Sm, anti-ds DNA
Rheumatoid arthritis	Symmetrical, small joints, deformity	Rheumatoid factor
Graves' disease	Hyperthyroid, extra-thyroidal signs	Anti-thyroid stimulating
Hashimoto's	Hypothyroid	Anti-thyroid peroxidase, anti-thyroglobulin
Myasthenia gravis	Skeletal muscle involvement Intermittent symptoms	Anti-acetylcholine receptor
Primary biliary cirrhosis	Middle-aged female Pruritus, high alkaline phosphatase	Anti-mitochondrial
Autoimmune hepatitis	Aminotransferase abn > alkaline phosphatase	Anti-smooth muscle
Sjögren syndrome	95% female Dry mouth and eyes	Anti-nuclear; rheumatoid factor
Scleroderma (systemic sclerosis)	Skin thickening; Pulmonary fibrosis Raynaud's Cardiorenal disease	Anti-nuclear, anti-Scl70

Blood Enzymes in Clinical Diagnosis

Serum enzyme levels are commonly measured in the diagnosis of disease. A brief description of their role in specific disorders will help you answer exam questions.

Serum Enzyme	Characteristic	Used in Diagnosis
Glucose-6 phosphate dehydrogenase	X-linked genetic deficiency	Infection, meds (e.g., primaquine) may trigger hemolysis
Angiotensin-converting enzyme	Found in lung, endothelium	Elevated in 50% of sarcoid
Alkaline phosphatase	Found in liver and bone	Intra- and extra-hepatic obstruction; bone disease
Gamma-glutamyl transpeptidase (GGTP)	In liver Not in bone	Cholestatic disease

(continued)

Serum Enzyme	Characteristic	Used in Diagnosis
Aminotransferases	In liver, skeletal muscle	Hepatocellular injury
Amylase	Pancreatic/salivary/	Pancreatic/GI /gyn/parotid disorders
Creatine kinase	Skeletal and cardiac muscle	CK-MM in myositis
	Brain	CK-MB in myocardial infarction

A classic question: Laboratory serum levels in a 77-year-old man show elevation of the alkaline phosphatase, but a normal gamma-glutamyl transpeptidase (GGTP) level. Which of the following is the most likely diagnosis? The answer will be bone disease (e.g., metastatic tumor in bone or Paget's disease of bone). In contrast, the serum alkaline phosphatase and GGTP levels will both be increased in cholestatic liver disease in which there is obstruction to bile flow.

Other Important, Selected Blood Diagnostic Tests

D-dimer is a degradation product of fibrin and, therefore, is used in the diagnosis of pulmonary embolism. D-dimer is of greater clinical significance when it is *normal*. If D-dimer by ELISA is normal, pulmonary embolism can be excluded with 95% accuracy.

Systemic arterial blood gas determinations define the acid-base status of the patient. Remember, in the patient with metabolic acidosis, always calculate the *anion gap*. Increased anion gap metabolic acidosis is characteristic of diabetic ketoacidosis, lactic acidosis, renal insufficiency, and poisoning due to salicylates, methanol, and ethylene glycol.

Brain natriuretic peptide (BNP) is released by myocardial cells in response to increased ventricular pressures. Therefore, in the patient who has dyspnea, BNP is used to differentiate between heart failure (cardiac) and pulmonary disease as the cause of the symptom.

Serologic tests for *Helicobacter pylori* are less accurate than fecal antigen immunoassay and C13 urea breath test.

A very important serum marker is alpha-fetoprotein. Alpha-fetoprotein is a serum marker for neural tube defect in the pregnant woman. It is elevated in 95% of males who have testicular germ cell gonadal tumors. In patients with cirrhosis, an increasing serum level of alpha-fetoprotein raises concern for hepatocellular carcinoma.

You are now able to answer many questions on PANCE and PANRE. These questions may ask you to select the serum enzyme that is most appropriate to order in a suspected condition. Alternatively, the question stem may give you the enzyme value and then ask you the most likely diagnosis.

Imaging Studies

In cardiology, the echocardiogram plays a key role in diagnosis. In addition to demonstrating chamber volume, valvular function, and wall thickness, from the echocardiogram one can determine aortic root dimension, left ventricular ejection fraction, and evidence of aorta dissection, or pericardial tamponade. Consequently, many PANCE and PANRE questions may address the role of echocardiography in the diagnosis of chronic and acute cardiac disorders.

When you know the previous facts, you are able to answer many questions that relate to the laboratory or imaging studies that are performed in clinical diagnosis.

FORMULATING MOST LIKELY DIAGNOSIS

Making the diagnosis forces the test candidate to integrate the elements of history, physical examination, and laboratory/imaging studies. **Essentials** and **Answers to Essentials** sections of this book are designed to help you link these factors in formulating the most likely diagnosis.

One clinical example: A 54-year-old woman has a 3-month history of progressive nausea and an 8-pound weight loss. Sitting blood pressure is 104/68 mm Hg and standing pressure 82/53 mm Hg. Examination shows hyperpigmentation of the skin creases. Serum sodium concentration is 124 mEq/L. Which of the following is the most likely diagnosis? The symptoms, orthostatic hypotension, physical examination sign, and laboratory abnormality, when linked together, make the most likely diagnosis chronic adrenal insufficiency.

When reading a test question, try to think of the one disease that will represent the sum of symptoms, vital signs, physical examination signs, and diagnostic testing.

PANCE and PANRE examinations will determine whether you know the most likely infecting organism in the patient who has a specific disease or exposure. Here are examples:

Underlying Disease/Exposure	Likely Infecting Organism(s)
Sickle cell anemia	Encapsulated bacteria, esp. *Pneumococcus*
Cystic fibrosis	*Staphylococcus* *Pseudomonas*
Intravenous drug abuser	*Staphylococcus aureus*
Lung abscess	Anaerobic bacteria (e.g., *Fusiform bacilli*)
Contaminated water in showers	*Legionella pneumophila*
Swimming pools	*Cryptosporidium*

PHARMACEUTICAL THERAPEUTICS/CLINICAL INTERVENTION

These two tasks are interweaved because they represent management of the patient. The test candidate must know the actions of a medication, its clinical indications and contraindications, and important drug interactions. Here are some important examples:

Medicine	Clinical Intervention
Labetalol	Hemodynamic effects of cocaine
Aspirin	Primary and secondary prevention of atherosclerotic events
Beta-adrenergic blockers	Prevention of recurrent myocardial infarction; Used in therapy of *chronic* systolic heart failure (HF), but not in *acute* HF
Warfarin	Paroxysmal or chronic atrial fibrillation Mechanical heart valves

In selecting the preferred medication in a patient's therapy, you must be aware of two very important factors, namely, the patient's co-existing disease and the patient's present medication. Here are a few examples:

Avoid niacin in the patient with dyslipidemia who has gout, because niacin elevates serum uric acid concentration.

Avoid a thiazide diuretic in the patient with hypertension who has hyperuricemia, because thiazides elevate serum uric acid concentration and may precipitate a gout attack.

Avoid beta-adrenergic blockers in the patient who has obstructive lung disease or peripheral claudication, because beta blockers may exacerbate the pulmonary or extremity symptoms.

In the patient who takes warfarin therapy, remember that aspirin, acetaminophen, cephalosporins, erythromycin, omeprazole, influenza virus, and macrolide antibiotics (a partial list) increase warfarin's effect. Oppositely, nafcillin, haloperidol, vitamin K, and oral contraceptives decrease the warfarin effect.

HEALTH MAINTENANCE

Immunizations

Immunizations are important in prevention of communicable disease. You must know the immunization schedule for infants and small children.

Vaccine	Recommended for Those Persons
Meningococcal	College students living in dormitories
Pneumococcal	All > 65 years Younger persons having immunocompromised state Metabolic, liver, and cardiopulmonary diseases Alcohol abuse Sickle cell patients
Influenza	*Live* vaccine for healthy persons 5 to 49 years of age *Inactive* vaccine for persons :50 years Those with metabolic and cardiopulmonary diseases, immunocompromised persons Residents in chronic care facilities Women who will become pregnant during flu season Health-care workers

Complications of Disease State

Here are typical questions that will determine your knowledge of a disease complication.

Question 1: A 64-year-old man has chronic, severe heartburn due to gastro-esophageal reflux. He is at increased risk for which of the following? The answer is Barrett's esophagus.

Question 2: A 64-year-old man who has Barrett's esophagus would be expected to show which of the following histologic changes upon esophageal biopsy? The answer is columnar epithelium.

Question 3: A patient with Barrett's esophagus is at increased risk to develop which of the following? The answer is adenocarcinoma of the esophagus.

Here are two questions that determine whether you know the complications of pathophysiologic states.

Patients who have cardiac disorders characterized by increased ventricular preload are at risk to develop which of the following? The answer is systolic heart failure.

Patients who have cardiac disorders characterized by increased ventricular afterload are at risk to develop which of the following? The answer is diastolic heart failure.

Counseling

You should expect questions that will determine your knowledge in counseling. Here are some important examples of counseling that would make appropriate questions:

Patient	Counseling
Woman taking ACE inhibitor	Avoid pregnancy
Woman taking lithium	Avoid pregnancy Medication should be taken with meals
Any patient taking lithium	Thiazide increases lithium blood level
Marfan's syndrome	Avoid contact sports
Hypertensive patient	Lose weight if obese Restrict salt and alcohol intake Aerobic activity Low saturated-fat diet

Parents of infants and small children properly have health concerns over their children's development. "What should my child be able to do at 6 months . . . at 12 months?" You must know normal language and motor development milestones in infants and small children.

"My daughter has a stomach ache after drinking milk. Is it an allergy?" You must know that eggs, milk, wheat, peanuts, and soy are common allergens in young children. However, in older children and adolescents, fish, shellfish, and nuts are common allergens.

Index

A

Abdominal pain, diagnostic test for, 28, 104–105
Abruptio placentae, 209
Acanthamoeba keratitis, 59
Acanthosis nigricans
    conditions associated with, 10, 57
    gastric adenocarcinoma and, 166
Acetaminophen
    osteoarthritis, dosage for, 181
    toxicity risk, increase in, 18, 79
Acetylcholine receptor antibody, 30, 109
Acquired immune deficiency syndrome (AIDS)
    HIV developing into, 207
    infection, abnormality causing, 33, 117–118
    infection, prophylaxis against, 34, 119
Acromegaly, 94–95
Acute bacterial prostatitis, *Pseudomonas* causing, 216
Acute cholecystitis, symptoms of, 149
Acute coronary syndrome, 27, 100–101
Acute glomerulonephritis, 65, 169
Acute myocardial infarction
    medication contraindicated for, 12
    preferred medication for, 12
Acute pancreatitis, 82, 183, 230
Acute pericarditis, 7
    conditions associated with, 52
Acute thoracic dissection of aorta
    complication from, 11, 62
    symptoms of, 158
    tests for, 6, 51
Addison's disease
    characteristics of, 16, 73
    cosyntropin stimulation test for, 152
Adenocarcinoma of pancreas, symptoms of, 216
Adenocarcinoma of stomach, symptoms of, 155
Adrenal insufficiency
    plasma adrenocorticotropin level, elevated, 169
    symptoms of, 170
Afterload, 241
Agranulocytosis, 192
Alcohol
    acetaminophen toxicity, 79
    delirium tremens from, 36, 126–127
    gout and, 79–80
    macrocytosis and, 65–66
    pain in left great toe, therapy for, 19
    rosacea rash, worsening of, 178
Alcohol abuse
    consequence of, 16, 72
    hepatitis, laboratory values suggesting, 199
    macrocytosis and, 169
    therapeutic measures for, 145
    vomiting blood, treatment for, 148

Alcoholic hallucinosis, 211
Alkaline phosphatase, 247
Allergen, 9
Allergic rhinitis, 67, 69
Allopurinol, 157
Alpha-fetoprotein
    germ cell testicular tumor, 206
    hepatocellular carcinoma, 206
    importance of, 248
    levels in hepatocellular carcinoma, 152, 173
Alpha-glucosidase inhibitor, 211
Amantadine, 30, 108
Amaurosis fugax, 153
Aminotransferase, 248
Amiodarone, 72
Amylase
    characteristics and uses of, 248
    elevation of, cause of, 20
Amyloidosis, 94–95
Amyotrophic lateral sclerosis, fasciculation, 203
Anginal equivalent, symptoms of, 147
Angina pectoris
    characteristics of, 244–245
    pneumococcal vaccination for, 17
    verapamil as treatment for, 171
Angiotensin-converting enzyme, 157
Angiotensin-converting enzyme inhibitor therapy
    asthmatic tolerating, 186
    characteristics and uses of, 247
    disease treated with, 24, 52, 91
    hypertension, as treatment for, 175
    indications for, 7
    nephrotic syndrome, 203
    nonproductive cough, 89–90
    pregnancy and, 174, 185
    proteinuria, as treatment for, 150
Anion gap metabolic acidosis, end-stage renal disease, 195
Ankle deep tendon reflex, absence of, 39, 136–137
Annular lesion, 19
    cause of, 81
Anomalous coronary artery, 48
Anorectal manometry, symptoms of, 155
Anthrax, 21, 85
Anti-acetylcholine, myasthenia gravis, 202
Antibody formation, 13
    disease associated with, 66–67
Anti-phospholipid antibody, 209
Antiphospholipid antibody syndrome, 197, 234
Anti–thyroid-stimulating hormone receptor antibodies, 194

253

Aorta
  coarctation of, 171, 225
  complication of acute dissection of, 11
  dissection of, risk factors, 38, 131–132
  tests for acute thoracic dissection of, 6, 51
Aorta dissection, 245
Aortic valve regurgitation, 25, 94
Aortic valve stenosis, 242
Arterial thrombosis, 23
Arteriovenous fistula, 25, 93
  symptoms of, 191
Ascariasis, 38, 131
Ascending cholangitis, 198
Ascites
  disorder associated with, 22, 87
  hepatic encephalopathy, 35, 122
  portal hypertension, 190
Aseptic meningitis, infectious mononucleosis and, 156
Aspirin, asthma and, 69
Asthma
  angiotensin-converting enzyme inhibitor therapy and, 186
  aspirin and, 69
  low humidity in air cabin, 212
Atherosclerosis, 48
  risk factor for, 245
Atherosclerotic stenosis
  symptom of, 9, 55–56
Ativan (sublingual lorazepam), 184
Atrial septal defect, 41, 138
Atrioventricular conduction
  medication slowing, 50
  medications slowing, 6
Attention-deficit hyperactivity disorder, 9
  characteristics of, 56
Autoimmune disease, 246
Autoimmune hepatitis, 247
Autonomic insufficiency
  orthostatic hypotension, cause of, 163
  symptoms of, 150, 208
  syncope, cause of, 242–243
Aviation Medical Assistance Act of 1998, 37, 128
Azithromycin, indication for, 201

B

Bacteremia, 80
Bacterial vaginosis, symptoms of, 215
Bacteriuria, 134–135
Benzodiazepine anti-anxiety medicine, 78
Beriberi, 25, 94
Beta-adrenergic blocker, 63
  hypoglycemia, causing, 114
Betamethasone with clotrimazole (Lotrisone), 175
Bicuspid aortic valve, 171, 225
  aortic stenosis, 172
Biliary cirrhosis, 52
Biliary cirrhosis, anti-mitochondrial antibodies, 199
Bilirubin
  increase in, 4
  jaundice and, 47
Binocular diplopia, 61
Bioterrorist attack, 21
  high-risk infectious diseases from, 85
Bismuth poisoning, 46
Bisphosphonate, 158
Blood diagnostics, 248
Blood pressure
  hydrochlorothiazide, checking while taking, 181
  secondary cause of elevation in, 14, 69–70
  thiazide therapy for, 162
Blood urea nitrogen (BUN), 20, 82–83
Blurred vision
  cataracts, as symptom of, 155
  duplex carotid artery ultrasound, 158
Brain natriuretic peptide (BNP), 248
Bronchiectasis, 165
Bronchitis, chronic, 8

C

Calcium, 158
Calf
  injury, cause of pain in diabetic, 25, 93
  pain from malignancy, 27, 100
Campylobacter jejuni, 190
Cancer, clubbing and, 70
Candida, 34, 119
Captopril
  contraindication for, 205
  hypertension, as treatment for, 175
  indication for, 185
Carbohydrate, alpha-glucosidase inhibitor, 211
Carbon monoxide
  decreased diffusing capacity, 160, 221
  poisoning, diagnostic test for, 38, 133
  poisoning, treatment for, 215
Carcinoma
  human papillomavirus causing, 126
  iron deficiency, cause of, 115
Cardiac function, overview of, 241–242
Carotid artery stenosis
  symptoms of, 9
  unilateral, 165, 223
Carpal tunnel syndrome
  cause of, 25, 94–95
  serum thyroid-stimulating hormone level, 195
Cataract
  Prednisone and formation of, 166
  symptoms of, 155
Ceftriaxone, 215
Celebrex, myocardial infarction risk, 188
Celiac disease
  gastrointestinal absorption of iron, decreased, 205
  iron deficiency, cause of, 115
Central cranial nerve VII palsy, 168
  peripheral cranial nerve VII palsy, differentiating, 224
Central venous pressure, 6
  conditions increasing, 51
Central vertigo, 38, 132
Cerebellar degeneration, 7, 53–54

Cerebral aneurysm
    congenital disorder associated with, 11, 61–62
    cranial nerve palsy, causing, 72
    diplopia and, 61
Cesarean delivery, 28, 103–104
Chest, anterior pain, 27
Chlorpromazine (Thorazine), causing jaundice, 198
Cholera, hypokalemia and, 156
Chronic bronchitis
    pulmonary fibrosis, differentiating, 166, 224
    typical findings complicated by right heart failure, 8
Chronic obstructive lung disease, 180
Chronic primary adrenal insufficiency, 16
    characteristics of, 73
Chronic stable angina pectoris, 17
Ciprofloxacin, 216
Cirrhosis
    ascites formation and, 87
    complications from, 6, 50
    hepatic encephalopathy, cause of, 35, 122
    vomiting blood, treatment for, 148
Clarithromycin, 186
Clonidine, 174
Clubbing (of fingers and toes)
    Crohn's disease, 49
    disorder associated with, 15, 70, 245–246
Cocaine
    cardiovascular complications from, 5, 48–49
    verapamil for countering effects of, 147
Coccidioidomycosis, 44
    diagnostic test for, 140–141
Colon cancer, ulcerative colitis and, 196
Community acquired pneumonia, 21, 84
Complete blood count, 246
Condylomata acuminata, 126
Confusion, 125–126
Constrictive pericarditis
    increased central pressure in, 6, 51
    symptoms of, 148
Contact lens
    complication from, 10, 59
    corneal ulceration risk, 156
    extended wear, 157, 221
Corneal ulceration, risk of, 156
Coronary artery spasm, 48
Cor pulmonale
    cause of, 242
    pathophysiologic abnormality in, 18, 77
    symptoms of, 178
Cosyntropin stimulation test, 152
Cough
    blood with, cause in smoker, 24
    nonproductive, medication causing, 24
Counseling, 251
Cranial nerve III mononeuropathy, 34, 119–120
Cranial nerve palsy, 15
    diseases causing, 71–72
Cranial nerve V function, 172
Cranial nerve VII, 10
    maneuver for testing function, 59

C-reactive protein, 8
    increased level of, 54
Creatine kinase, 248
Crohn's disease
    acute cholecystitis, symptoms, 149
    hypertrophic osteoarthropathy and, 162
    manifestation of, 5, 49
    vitamin B_{12}, need for, 162
    vitamin B_{12} deficiency and, 66
Cryptosporidium, symptoms of, 191
Cushing's disease, 245
Cyclooxygenase 2 (COX 2), 23
    arterial thrombosis, increasing risk of, 87–88
Cystic fibrosis
    bronchiectasis as complication of, 165
    pneumonia, *pseudomonas aeruginosa* causing, 164
Cystic fibrosis (CF), 69
Cystic fibrosis (CF), clubbing, 70
Cystitis, 65

D
Deep vein thrombosis, 24, 92–93
    nephrotic syndrome and, 202
    oral contraception, contraindication for, 37, 129
    platelet count, 165
    progestin-only contraceptive, 204
    squamous cell carcinoma of lung, 27, 100
Dehydration, 35, 124–125
Delirium tremens, 36, 126–127
    alcoholic hallucinosis, differentiating, 211
    thiamine for, 211
Dementia
    alcohol abuse and, 145
    cause of, 4, 45–46
Depression, 46
Diabetes
    calf injury, cause of pain, 25
    diplopia,, 33
    gastroparesis, indication of, 22, 87
Diabetes insipidus, 210
Diabetes mellitus
    foot drop/peroneal nerve palsy, 208
    gestational, exercise and, 204
    sudden cardiac arrest, risk of, 208
Diabetes mellitus, type 1
    autoimmune destruction of pancreatic B cells, 180
    gastroparesis, indication of, 188
    glucagon, elevated levels of, 176
    HLA-DR3 gene, 183
    nocturnal diarrhea, 208
Diabetes mellitus, type 2
    cranial nerve palsy, causing, 71–72
    glyburide therapy during pregnancy, 205
    hyperphosphatemia, 35, 122–123
    hypoglycemia, medication causing, 32, 114
    insulin resistance, 183, 229
    metformin, contraindication for, 200, 235
    pathophysiologic abnormality in, 20, 83
    proteinuria and, treatment for, 150
    symptoms of, 158, 164
    therapy, preferred initial, 30, 107–108

therapy for, 37, 127–128
thiazolidinediones, 212
Diabetic autonomic neuropathy (DAN), 34, 120
Diabetic ketoacidosis, 29
　IV solution for, 107
Diabetic nephropathy
　anion gap metabolic acidosis, increased, 195
　condition least likely found with, 30, 109–110
Diagnosis, formulation of, 249
Diarrhea
　bloody, flexible sigmoidoscopy for, 194
　bloody, NSAID causing in inflammatory colitis, 192
　cholera and hypokalemia, 156
　nocturnal, 208
　organisms causing, 26, 97–98
Diastolic heart failure (DHF), 4, 45
　cause of, 241–242
　symptoms of, 146
Diffusion impairment, 243–244
Digoxin, 50
　toxicity, hypokalemia and, 159
　toxicity risk, increase in, 12, 64
　ventricular rate, controlling, 145
Dilated cardiomyopathy, 173
Diltiazem, 173
Diplopia
　cause of, 11, 61
　diabetic exhibiting, 34, 119–120
Disease, complications of, 250–251
Diverticulosis, 184, 230
Doxazosin, hypotension risk, 214
Dubin-Johnson syndrome, 47
Dumping syndrome, 126, 210
Dyslipidemia, niacin therapy for, 151, 219
Dysmenorrhea, 29, 104–105
　ibuprofen for, 199
Dysmetria, 38, 132
Dysphagia, 12
　esophageal motility disorder, 63
Dyspnea, 17
　blood diagnostic studies for, 75

E

Echocardiogram, role of, 248
Eclampsia, 197, 234
Ectopic adrenocorticotrophic hormone (ACTH), 164
Ectopic pregnancy
　bipolar coagulation sterilization, 197
　serum amylase, elevation of, 82
　testing for, 28, 102
Endocarditis, 69
　clubbing and, 70
　night sweats, 110
Endocarditis prophylaxis
　indication for, 19, 80
　mechanical heart valve in aortic position, 182
　mitral valve prolapse, as contraindication for, 179
Endoscopic retrograde cholangiography, 28, 104–105

Endothelial dysfunction, preeclampsia and, 197
End-stage renal disease
　anion gap metabolic acidosis, increased, 195
　hyperphosphatemia, 35, 122–123
Enteritis, 190
Enterotoxigenic *Escherichia coli*, 97–98
Enzyme labeled immunosorbent assay (ELISA), 118, 157
Eosinophil, 14
　nasal secretions, finding in, 67
Eosinophilia, 131
Epidural blood patch, 193
Erythema infectiosum, symptoms of, 207
Erythema migrans, 166
Escherichia coli, 39, 135–136, 216
Esophagitis, 7, 53
Exophthalmos, 26, 95–96
Extensor Babinski's response, 207
Extravascular hemolysis, 47, 205

F

Facial roseola, 177
Fainting
　heightening vagal tone, 154
　with long QT interval, 16
　See also Syncope
　serum creatine kinase and troponin levels, 153
Fasciculation, 203
Ferritin, 205
Fluoroquinolone
　risk factor of, 23, 89
　as treatment for pyuria/bacteriuria, 39, 134–135
Focal glomerulosclerosis, oral angiotensin-converting enzyme inhibitor, 202
Folic acid deficiency anemia, 161
Folliculitis, 43, 184
Foot drop, diabetes mellitus, 208

G

G-6 PD (Glucose-6 phosphate dehydrogenase) deficiency, 47
Gamma-glutamyl transpeptidase (GGTP), 247
Gastrectomy
　fever, cause of, 31, 111–112
　intrinsic factor production, lack of, 162
Gastric achlorhydria, 169
Gastric adenocarcinoma
　acanthosis nigricans, 166
　risk factor for, 21, 84–85
Gastroesophageal reflux, 99–100
　chocolate ice cream, 195
　symptoms of, 26, 196
Gastroparesis
　indication in diabetic patient, 22, 87, 188
　nuclear scintigraphy after radioactive-labeled meal, 189
Genetic transmission, 244–245
Germ cell testicular tumor, Alpha-fetoprotein levels, 206
Gestational hypertension, 196, 234
Giardia, 97–98

Giardia lamblia
   Campylobacter jejuni differentiating from, 190
   symptoms of, 190
Gilbert's disease, 47
Glomerulonephritis, acute, 65
Glucose-6 phosphate dehydrogenase deficiency, 4
   characteristics and uses of, 247
   symptoms of, 146
Glyburide, 32, 114
   pregnancy and, 205
Gonococcal urethritis, ceftriaxone for, 215
Gout, 79–80
   niacin, 147
   treatment for, 182, 229
Gram-negative bacteremia, 194, 233
Graves' disease
   anti–thyroid-stimulating hormone receptor antibodies, 194
   characteristics and antibodies of, 247
   exophthalmos, 95–96
   hyperthyroidism, differentiating, 202
   iron deficiency, cause of, 115
Groin, diagnostic test for burning in, 40, 137
Guillain-Barré syndrome, 96–97

H

Haloperidol (Haldol), 77, 179
Hashimoto's, 247
Hay fever, 171, 225
Headache, life-threatening, 39, 134
Heartburn, Ranitidine for, 196
Heart failure, 6, 45
   cause of, 35, 55, 123–124
   diastolic, 4
   high cardiac output, cause of, 25
   increased central pressure in, 51
   symptoms of, 153
   ventricular wall stretching, 164
Heart murmur, 41, 138
Heart valve, mechanical prosthetic
   endocarditis prophylaxis, indication for, 19
Helicobacter pylori gastritis, 21, 84–85
   iron deficiency, cause of, 115
   therapy agents not used with, 29, 106–107
Helicobacter pylori infection, 29
   diagnostic test for, 106
Hematuria
   condition associated with, 13
   conditions associated with, 65
Hemolysis
   increased serum bilirubin levels, 47
   laboratory values from, 5, 49
Hemolytic anemia
   symptoms of, 198
Hemorrhaging
   diabetes insipidus, 210
   extensive, initial treatment for, 22, 85–86
Henoch-Schönlein purpura, 65
   symptoms of, 160
Heparin therapy
   platelet count, 165

Hepatic encephalopathy (HE)
   cause of, 35, 122
   hypokalemia precipitating, 238
Hepatitis, chronic active, 37, 129
Hepatitis B serologic markers
   immunity to, 198
   indications from, 28, 102–103
Hepatobiliary disease, 47
Hepatocellular carcinoma
   alpha-fetoprotein levels in, 152, 173, 206
Hereditary spherocytosis
   splenectomy recommendations, 34, 122
Herpes zoster
   characteristics of, 23, 88–89
   vaccine recommendations, 75
High blood pressure
   management during pregnancy, 32
High cardiac output heart failure, 25, 93–94
Hirschsprung's disease
   abnormal findings in infant with, 9, 56–57
HLA-DR3 gene, 183
Hodgkin's disease
   night sweats, 110
   symptoms of, 202
Human immunodeficiency virus (HIV), 117–118
   AIDS, developing into, 207
Human papillomavirus (HPV)
   manifestation of, 36, 126
   symptoms of, 211
Hydrocephalus, normal pressure, 146
Hydrochlorothiazide
   hypertension, as treatment for, 176
   lithium therapy and, 165
Hyperglycemia
   conditions associated with, 38, 130
   medications causing, 9, 57
Hyperkalemia
   serum potassium levels, 246
   therapeutic intervention for, 10, 58
Hypernatremia, 124–125
Hypersegmented neutrophils, pernicious anemia and, 160
Hypertension
   angiotensin-converting enzyme inhibitor therapy, 175
   Captopril as treatment for, 175
   cause of, 21
   clonidine, discontinuing, 174
   hydrochlorothiazide as treatment for, 176, 181
   medication causing, 38, 130–131
   medication for, 17, 21, 75–76
   pheochromocytoma, as symptom of, 152
   polycystic kidney disease, 168
   secondary cause of, 14, 69–70
   thiazide and leg claudication, 182
Hyperthyroidism, 25, 93
   exophthalmos and, 26, 95–96
   Graves' disease, differentiating, 202
   serum thyroid-stimulating hormone level, 196
   symptoms of, 163, 192
Hypertriglyceridemia, 37, 129

Hypertrophic cardiomyopathy, 244
Hypertrophic obstructive cardiomyopathy
  syncope, cause of, 242–243
Hypertrophic obstructive cardiomyopathy,
  symptoms of, 147
Hypertrophic osteoarthropathy
  Crohn's disease and, 162
Hypertrophic pyloric stenosis (HPS), 127
Hypertrophy cardiomyopathy
  medication for, 145
Hyperuricemic nephropathy
  prophylactic allopurinol for prevention of, 167
Hypoglycemia
  manifestation of, 36, 125–126
  medication causing in diabetes mellitus type 2, 32
  seizure, as cause of, 210
Hypokalemia
  cause of, 10, 57–58
  cholera and diarrhea, 156
  conditions associated with, 30
  digoxin toxicity and, 159
  hepatic encephalopathy (HE), 238
  loop diuretic therapy, 108
  serum potassium levels, 246
Hypomagnesemia
  QT interval, prolongation of, 167
Hyponatremia
  excess water as cause of, 210
  heart failure, as cause of, 35, 123–124
  small cell carcinoma and SIADH, 188
Hypotension
  doxazosin causing, 214
Hypotension, orthostatic
  cause of, 7
  medication causing, 14
Hypothyroidism
  carpal tunnel syndrome, 94–95
  macrocytosis and, 65–66
  medication causing, 15, 72
  pernicious anemia and, 169
  symptoms of, 246
Hypoventilation, 243–244
Hypovolemia
  orthostatic hypotension, 184, 230
  signs of, 22, 86, 163
Hypoxemia, cause of, 243–244

I
Idiopathic diffuse pulmonary fibrosis, 160, 221
Idiopathic thrombocytopenia purpura, 69
Idiopathic thrombocytopenic purpura, 37, 128–129
Imaging studies, 248
Immunization, 250
Impetigo planus, 77
Indomethacin, 181, 229
Infantile hypertrophic pyloric stenosis (IHPS), 127
Infectious, noninflammatory diarrhea
  organism causing, 26
Infectious mononucleosis
  aseptic meningitis and, 156
  complication from, 10, 58–59
  saliva, contagiousness of, 177, 228
  streptococcus and, 177
  symptoms of, 80–81
Influenza
  live attenuated vaccine, recommendation for, 192, 232
  medication not recommended for, 30, 108
Insulin
  resistance to, 20, 83, 183, 229
Intention tremor
  cause of, 7, 53–54
Interstitial fibrosis
  arterial blood values for, 159
Intranasal beclomethasone, 171, 225
Intravascular hemolysis, 47
  blood in urine, 206
  extravascular hemolysis, differentiating, 205
  iron deficiency, cause of, 115
Intravenous immune globulin
  as treatment for, 37, 128–129
Intrinsic factor production, 162
Iron deficiency
  cause of, 33, 115–116
  gastrointestinal absorption in celiac patient, 205
  symptoms of, 206
Irritable bowel syndrome
  travelers' diarrhea, 191
Isosorbide dinitrate, 76

J
Jaundice
  asymptomatic, 146
  cause of, 4, 47
  Chlorpromazine (Thorazine) as causative agent, 198
  disease associated with, 245–246
  increase in bilirubin, 4

K
Kawasaki disease, 37, 128–129
  coronary artery aneurysm, 212
  intravenous immune globulin and aspirin, 212
Keratitis, 59

L
Lactic acid, production of, 194
Lactic acidosis, metformin increasing risk
  of, 200
Lactulose enema, 209, 238
Left ventricular hypertrophy, 48
Leg claudication
  thiazide and hypertension, 182
Legionnaires' disease
  hotel as source, 186
  symptoms of, 187
Lichen planus, 77
  symptoms of, 177
Lidocaine, myocardial infarction, 201
Lightheadedness, cause of, 150
Lisinopril, 214

Lithium therapy
  hydrochlorothiazide during, 165
  hypothyroidism as side effect, 72
  pregnancy and, 155, 165
  side effect of, 8, 55
  thyroid function values, 153
Live attenuated influenza vaccine
  recommendation for, 25, 95, 192, 232
Liver
  cirrhosis of, 6, 50
  failure of, 37, 129
  function testing, 181
Liver disease, 246
Long QT interval
  fainting, as cause of, 16, 73, 168
Loop diuretic therapy, 30, 108
Lumbar puncture
  epidural blood patch for headache, 193
  indication for, 26, 96–97
  subarachnoid hemorrhage, 193
Lung cancer, 245
Lyme disease
  cranial nerve palsy, causing, 71
  erythema migrans, 166
Lymphadenopathy
  cause of, 19
Lymphoma
  night sweats, 110

M

Macrocytosis
  alcohol abuse and, 169
  cause of, 13, 65–66
Macrolide, symptoms of, 211
Malarial prophylaxis, 146
Malar rash
  disease associated with, 246
Marfan's syndrome, 244, 245
Mechanical prosthetic heart valve
  endocarditis prophylaxis, indication for, 19
Mediterranean diet
  results of, 23, 89
Megaloblastic anemia
  intrinsic factor production, lack of, 162
  macrocytosis and, 65–66
Memory loss, normal pressure hydrocephalus, 146
Meningitis, 96–97
Meningococcal vaccine, 75
Meningococcemia, 69, 245
Menstruation
  panic disorder and, 174
Mesenteric infarction
  serum amylase, elevation of, 82
Metabolic acidosis, 25, 94
  laboratory determination for, 25
  lactic acid, production of, 194
Metabolic syndrome, 21, 83
  polycystic ovary syndrome, differentiating, 183, 229
Metformin, 30, 107–108
  lactic acidosis, risk of, 200
  peripheral arteriography/radiocontrast agent, 200

Methimazole, indication for, 195
Methotrexate
  liver function tests, 181
  recommendation with, 18, 78–79
Methylmalonic acid, 160
Metoprolol
  indication for, 167
  indications for, 161
Metronidazole gel, 177
Migraine, 165, 223, 243
Monocular diplopia, 61
Mononucleosis, infectious
  complication from, 10
  symptoms of, 80–81
Multiple sclerosis, 61, 96–97
Mumps
  serum amylase, elevation of, 82
Myasthenia gravis, 61
  anti-acetylcholine, 202
  antibodies to acetylcholine receptors, 109
  antibody formation and, 67
  characteristics and antibodies of, 247
  cranial nerve palsy, causing, 72
Myocardial infarction
  Celebrex, risk when taking, 188
  C-reactive protein, 54
  Lidocaine causing, 201
  medication contraindicated for, 12, 63
  medication for, 12, 63–64
  risk for recurrent, 151
  syncope, cause of, 54–55
Myocardial ischemia, 5, 48

N

Nails, pitting of, 174, 246
Nasal polyp
  disorder complicated by, 14, 69
  eosinophils in nasal secretions, 67
Nateglinide, 37, 127–128
Neisseria gonorrhoeae, 189
Nephrotic syndrome
  angiotensin-converting enzyme inhibitor therapy, 203
  deep vein thrombosis, 202
  diabetes, condition least likely found with, 30, 109–110
  in heroin addict, diagnosis, 31, 112–113
  increased central pressure in, 6, 51–52
  oral angiotensin-converting enzyme inhibitor, 202
  transudative pleural effusion, 188
Neural tube defect (NTD), 33, 116
Niacin therapy
  effects of, 151
  gout, contraindication for, 147
  orthostatic hypotension, causing, 68
  side effect of, 5, 48, 57
Nifedipine, 50
Night sweats, 31, 110
Nitroglycerin, 167
Non-Hodgkin's lymphoma
  night sweats, 110

260   Index

oral allopurinol for, 157
superior vena cava syndrome, development of, 172
symptoms of, 148
Nonproductive cough, 24
medication causing, 89
Nonsteroidal anti-inflammatory medicine (NSAID)
adverse effects of, 18, 52, 77
bloody diarrhea, 192
contraindication for, 214
as gout treatment, 79–80
hypertension, cause of, 38, 130–131
Normal pressure hydrocephalus, 146
Norovirus, 97–98
Nuclear scintigraphy after radioactive-labeled meal, 189

O

Oats, allergy to, 154
Obsessive-compulsive disorder, 22, 86
Octreotide, 148
Oculomotor palsy, 61
Ofloxacin, contraindication for, 189
Oral allopurinol, 157, 166
Oral contraceptive
contraindication for, absolute, 32, 113–114, 129
ovarian cancer, decreased risk of, 213
Orthostatic hypotension
autonomic insufficiency causing, 163
cause of, 7, 52–53
hypovolemia as sign of, 86, 184
medication causing, 14, 67–68
Parkinson's disease, 204
positional vertigo and presyncope, differentiating, 214
syncope, cause of, 54–55, 242–243
Osteoarthritis, 181
Osteopenia, 158
Osteoporosis, medication instructions for, 150, 218
Ovarian cancer, oral contraceptive and, 213

P

Paget's disease of bone
abnormal laboratory values with, 16, 74
laboratory values with, 172, 173
Palatal petechiae, 19
Pallor, 246
Palpitation
pheochromocytoma, as symptom of, 152
treatment for, 41, 138–139
Panic disorder
manifestation of, 22, 86
menstruation and, 174
sublingual lorazepam (Ativan), 184
Parkinson's disease
orthostatic hypotension, 204
symptoms of, 203
Parkinsonism, 31, 111
Paroxysmal supraventricular tachycardia, 168
Parvovirus, 33, 117
Pemphigus rash, 40, 137

Penicillin, spleen infarction, 209
Pericardial tamponade, 246
Pericarditis, acute, 7
conditions associated with, 52
Periorbital edema, 246
Peripheral cranial nerve VII palsy, 168
central cranial nerve VII palsy, differentiating, 224
Peripheral edema, 16, 74
Peripheral vertigo, 38, 132
Peritoneal carcinomatosis, 22, 87
Pernicious anemia
abnormal neurologic signs, 15, 71
folic acid deficiency anemia, differentiating from, 161
gastric achlorhydria and, 169
gastric adenocarcinoma, 21, 84–85
hypersegmented neutrophils, 160
hypothyroidism and, 169
methylmalonic acid, 160
vitamin B_{12} deficiency and, 66
Peroneal nerve palsy, diabetes mellitus, 208
Petechiae
disease associated with, 14, 68–69, 245–246
palatal, cause of, 19
Pheochromocytoma, 52, 152
Phlebitis, superficial, 25, 93
Phosphodiesterase 5 inhibitor, 177, 227
Placenta previa, 34, 121, 209
Plague, 21, 85
Plantar wart, 126
Plasma adrenocorticotropin level, elevation of, 169
Plasma glucose determination, 32
during pregnancy, Native Americans, 114
Plasma Nt-BNP, 164
Platelet, 165
Pleural effusion, 91–92
Pneumococcal vaccine, 17, 74–75, 207, 238
Pneumonia
cause of, 21, 84
with effusion, symptoms of, 187
Pseudomonas aeruginosa, 186
treatment for, 184, 230
Pneumonia Patient Outcomes Research Team (PORT), 24, 90–91
Polycystic kidney disease, 65, 244
hypertension as cause of, 168
Polycystic ovary syndrome, 183, 213, 229
Polycythemia rubra vera, 6, 51
Portal hypertension
ascites, as cause of, 190
spontaneous bacterial peritonitis, 190
Positional vertigo, 214
Potassium hydroxide preparation of scales, 176
Prednisone, 57, 166
Preeclampsia
eclampsia, differentiating from, 234
endothelial dysfunction, 197
gestational hypertension, differentiating from, 196
risk factor for, 28, 101–102
Pregnancy
angiotensin-converting enzyme inhibitor therapy, 174, 185

anti-phospholipid antibodies, 209
antiphospholipid antibody syndrome, 197, 234
   carpal tunnel syndrome, 94–95
   gestational diabetes, exercise and, 204
   glyburide therapy during, 205
   lithium therapy and, 155, 165
   plasma glucose determination in Native American, 32, 114
   preeclampsia, risk factors for, 28, 101–102
   rash during, 139–140, 139–140
   serial high blood pressure, management of, 32
   tingling in fingers, 193, 233
   transvaginal ultrasonography, 197
Preload, 241
Premenstrual dysmorphic disorder, 29, 106, 199
Presyncope, 214
Primary biliary cirrhosis
   characteristics and antibodies of, 247
   symptoms of, 149
Primary dysmenorrhea, 28
Primary hyperaldosteronism, 52
Primary parkinsonism, 31, 111
Prolactin, increased secretion of, 213
Prophylactic allopurinol
   hyperuricemic nephropathy prevention, 167
Propranolol, 32, 114
   tremor, treatment of, 151
Prostate, 39, 135–136
Prosthetic heart valve, mechanical
   endocarditis prophylaxis, indication for, 19
Proteinuria, treatment of, 150
Pruritus, 51–52
   cause of, 6
   lesion, 20
Pseudomonas, 216
Pseudomonas aeruginosa, 43, 164, 184, 186
Psoriasis, 81
   nail pitting, 174, 246
   symptoms of, 81–82
Psoriatic arthritis, 175
Psychotropic medicine, 18
   extrapyramidal adverse effects from, 77–78
Pulmonary edema
   medication contraindicated for, 12
   preferred medication for, 12
Pulmonary embolism
   laboratory value for excluding, 24, 92–93
   serum D-dimer as test for, 185
Pulmonary fibrosis, 166
   chronic bronchitis, differentiating, 224
Pulmonary hypertension
   symptoms of, 154
Pulmonary parenchymal disease, 242
Pulse pressure
   decreased arterial compliance, 162
   increase in, 15, 70–71
Pustular lesion, 17
   skin disorders causing, 76–77
Pyuria, 39

Q
QT interval, 167

R
Ranitidine, for heartburn, 196
Rash
   bilateral erythematous malar, cause of, 33, 117
   from hot bath, 43, 184
   pemphigus, 40, 137
   during pregnancy, 42, 139–140
   tinea versicolor, 42, 139
Reflex syncope, 242
Renal cell carcinoma, 65
Renal failure
   serum amylase, elevation of, 82
Renal hyperperfusion, 82–83
Renal insufficiency, nebulized albuterol for, 201
Respiratory syncytial virus, 21, 84
Restless leg syndrome (RLS), 116
Reversible dementia, 4, 46
Rheumatoid arthritis
   bisphosphonate for, 158
   carpal tunnel syndrome, 94–95
   characteristics and antibodies of, 247
   psoriatic arthritis, differentiating, 175
Right heart failure
   cause of, 8, 55
   symptoms of, 153
Ringworm, 175, 227
Rocky Mountain spotted fever, 69
Romberg test, 163
Rosacea, 76
Rosacea rash, 178
Rotavirus, 97–98

S
Sarcoidosis
   antibody formation and, 67
   arterial blood values for, 159
   cranial nerve palsy, causing, 71
   increased serum levels, 11, 60
Scabies, 77, 177, 228
Scleroderma
   characteristics and antibodies of, 247
   symptoms of, 156, 159
Secondary syphilis, 81
Seizure
   conditions precipitating, 35, 124
   hypoglycemia causing, 210
   as hypoglycemic manifestation, 125–126
   transient ischemic attack, differentiating, 210
   transient neurologic symptoms, 243
Selective serotonin reuptake inhibitor, 199
Serotonin syndrome, 78, 180
Sertraline (Zoloft), 78, 179
Serum alpha-fetoprotein, 33, 116
Serum amylase, 20, 82
Serum anti-nuclear antibody titer, 170, 225
Serum conjugated (direct) bilirubin, 4, 47

Serum creatine kinase, fainting and, 153
Serum D-dimer, 24, 92–93
   duplex ultrasound, omitting need for, 185
   pulmonary embolism, as test for, 185
Serum potassium, 246
Serum potassium concentration, cause for checking, 214
Serum thyroid-stimulating hormone level
   for carpal tunnel syndrome diagnosis, 195
   for hyperthyroidism diagnosis, 196
Serum unconjugated (indirect) bilirubin
   increase in, 4
Sexual dysfunction, 176
Sickle cell anemia, 209
Sick sinus syndrome, 54–55
Sildenafil, 17, 76
Sjögren's syndrome, 247
Skin disorder, 17
Small cell carcinoma of lung, 164
Smoking
   blood with cough, cause of, 24
SIDS, increased risk for, 204
Spider angiomata, 37, 129
   disease associated with, 246
Spleen infarction, penicillin for, 209
Splenectomy, 34
   recommendation for, 122
Spontaneous bacterial peritonitis, 190
Squamous cell carcinoma of lung
   deep vein thrombosis, 27, 100
   with effusion, 28, 91–92
St. John's wort, 179
Staphylococcal folliculitis, 184
Staphylococcus aureus, 97–98
Stomach, adenocarcinoma of, 155
Streptococcus, 177
Subarachnoid hemorrhage, 54–55, 96–97
   lumbar puncture for, 193
Subclavian steal syndrome
   percutaneous luminal angioplasty, 203
   symptoms of, 31, 112, 203
Sublingual lorazepam (Ativan), 184
Sudden infant death syndrome (SIDS)
   risk factor for, 32, 113
   smoking and, 204
Superficial phlebitis, 25, 93
Superior vena cava (SVC) syndrome, 51
   non-Hodgkin's lymphoma, 172
   symptoms of, 246
Sweating
   as hypoglycemic manifestation, 125–126
   pheochromocytoma, as symptom of, 152
Syncope
   cause of, 8, 54–55, 242–243
   Long QT interval syndrome, 168, 224
   verapamil, side effects of, 148, 178
   See also Fainting
Syphilis, 81
Systemic arterial blood gas, 248
Systemic arterial carboxyhemoglobin, 38, 133
Systemic hypertension, 242

Systemic lupus erythematosus (SLE)
   antibody formation and, 67
   characteristics and antibodies of, 247
   sunlight, 170
   symptoms of, 150, 246
   white blood count levels, 152
Systolic heart failure (SHF), 241–242

T
Testicular torsion, 39, 133–134
Tetracycline
   antacids and, 161
   considerations for using, 12, 62
Thallium stress cardiac testing, 171, 225
Thiazide, 182
Thiazolidinedione, 212
Thrombocytopenia, 68–69, 245
Thrombolytic therapy, 23, 88
Thyroid, 153
Thyroid-stimulating hormone, deficiency of, 146
Tinea barbae, 77
Tinea corporis, 81
Tinea versicolor, 42, 139
Tonsil, inflamed, 19
Torsion, 39, 133–134
Tourette's syndrome, symptoms of, 154
t-PA, contraindication for, 187
Transesophageal echocardiogram, 149, 161
Transient ischemic attack, 210, 243
Transient neurologic symptoms, 243
Transudative pleural effusion, 188
Travelers' diarrhea, irritable bowel syndrome and, 191
Tremor
   Parkinson's disease, 203
   propranolol, 151
Trichinellosis, 38, 131
Trichomonas vaginitis, strawberry cervix, 215
Trivalent inactivated influenza vaccine, 193, 233
Troponin, fainting and, 153
Tularemia, 21, 85
Tumor lysis syndrome
   elevated laboratory value from, 11, 60
   oral allopurinol for prevention of, 166

U
Ulcerative colitis
   colon cancer and, 196
   hydrocortisone foam enema, 194
   manifestation of, 26, 98–99
Unilateral carotid artery stenosis, 165, 223
Urinalysis, 33, 116–117

V
Vasculitis, 245
Vasomotor rhinitis, 69
Vasovagal reaction, 8, 54
Vegan diet, 66
Ventilation-perfusion mismatch, 243–244
Ventricular function, 241

Ventricular rate
  controlling, 145
  dilated cardiomyopathy, 173
  Diltiazem, 173
  verapamil, 172
Ventricular wall stretching, 164
Verapamil
  adverse effect of, 148
  angina pectoris, as treatment for, 171
  cocaine, countering effects of, 147
  edema, causing, 74
  gout, treatment for, 84
  hypertrophy cardiomyopathy, 145
  indication for, 13, 21, 64–65
  paroxysmal supraventricular tachycardia, 168
  syncope as side effect of, 178
  ventricular rate, controlling, 172

Vertigo, 38
  brain stem versus inner ear disease, 132
Vitamin B_{12}
  alcohol abuse, 145
  for Crohn's disease, 66, 162
  deficiency, cause of, 13, 66
  dementia and, 46
Vomiting
  blood, treatment for, 148
  in infant, cause of, 36, 127

W
Wernicke's encephalopathy, 61

Z
Zoster rash, 189, 232